WHAT THE BEAUTY WORLD SAYS ABOUT ALISON

'Alison is a beauty industry powerhouse. Working with her was always educational, inspiring – and fun!' – Lulu

'I have met many beauty experts and none have impressed me more than Alison Young. Her expertise is second-to-none.' – Saira Kahn

'Alison is the real deal – someone who's had no cosmetic work so her readers know they're getting honest, expert, tried-and-trusted beauty advice.' – Elsa McAlonan, Beauty Columnist at the *Daily Mail*

'An amazingly knowledgeable therapist who really understands the science of skin and what skincare works. She's the queen of skincare!' – Oriele Frank, co-founder of Elemis

'Takes the complicated world of beauty and makes it user-friendly for all.' – Ruby Hammer, MBE, make-up artist and brand founder

'One of the most trusted voices in the industry.' – Lesley Thomas, Beauty Editor at *The Times*

'Alison is like a walking beauty encyclopaedia and stalwart of the industry. What she doesn't know probably isn't worth knowing.' – Edwina Ings-Chambers, Beauty Director at *You Magazine*

WHAT ALISON'S SOCIAL MEDIA FOLLOWERS SAY ABOUT HER

'Simply invaluable . . . a voice that can be relied upon to give helpful, clear advice alongside motivation and encouragement, with the experience and knowledge to back it up.'

'You made truly excellent skincare and routines accessible for all, irrespective of budget!'

'At 58 I have the best skin ever and I'm always complimented – thank you, thank you, thank you!'

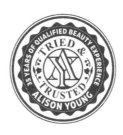

Born in the north of England and now living in the south, **Alison Young** is globally recognised as one of the most experienced, qualified professionals in the world of beauty. Alison won an 'Amazing Woman' Award from *Woman & Home* and CEW Awards, recognising her outstanding contribution to the industry. She is hugely respected and trusted by brand owners, CEOs, PRs, marketeers and, most importantly, her core fan base of real people at home.

During her 35 years' industry experience, Alison had advanced training as a beauty therapist and make-up artist, counting A-listers and royalty among her clientele, before becoming the UK's youngest ever Head of Training at Clarins. Since then, Alison has helped thousands of clients in person and trained countless other professionals, as well as designing treatments, training and strategy for numerous brands. Today, Alison splits her time between advisory roles for labs, brands and retailers, and her media work across TV, radio and social media. At QVC, where she first brought professional beauty into people's living rooms 29 years ago, she is watched by millions and has helped turn brands such as Molton Brown, Liz Earle and Elemis into household names.

THE
Beauty
Insider

ALISON
YOUNG

**EFFORTLESS SKINCARE
AND BEAUTY ADVICE
THAT WORKS**

CONTENTS

Introduction

"

Everywhere I go, I'm asked for beauty advice

Everywhere I go, I'm asked for beauty advice. I'm a walking, talking beauty consultant. I get asked questions in petrol stations. In A & E. In supermarkets. On ski lifts, where I'm wearing top-to-toe neoprene with not a visible square inch of skin, but someone recognises my voice and immediately shares a beauty challenge they'd like me to help with. It's easy to see what the answer means to them.

I might be paying for shopping and someone will look at my hands and go, 'I know those hands' (because they've seen me demoing on TV), then ask me a question. Once, coming round from an anaesthetic, I found the nurses looking at my hands, commenting on my manicure. Another time, in an ambulance, I had a medic jabbing me in the backside while asking, 'Are beauty products really that good?' So this book is for him. And for the thousands of other people who contact me for my online Q&A sessions, or my Instagram and Facebook Lives, wanting beauty answers. And the countless other people I meet who want to know more about the fascinating world of beauty I am lucky enough to work in, with its countless products – and its tons of confusion.

The beauty world, in reality, isn't about vanity. It's about wellbeing. Wanting glowing skin or wearing nice make-up or having a great haircut is actually about self-care. For most of us, the minutes we spend in a locked bathroom each morning and evening may be the only time we get to do something purely for ourselves, all day long.

Quite a chunk of my early life was spent travelling round the country visiting department stores with my dad, getting my first insights into shops and listening to customers; he worked his way up from shop assistant to director of House of Fraser. But my understanding of how our skin, in particular, is inextricably linked with our wellbeing, actually began when I was a very tiny child, covered in eczema. As a baby, I'd have my hands bandaged so that I couldn't scratch myself. But my clever mother, decades ahead of her time, figured out what worked to ease my suffering. She only dressed me in cotton, and if we travelled on public transport I'd sit on a tea towel, so the upholstery couldn't irritate my skin. She worked out that foaming products made it worse, long before that was understood by the medical profession.

As I grew into a young adult, I was left with scarring and pigmentation where I'd literally gouged out my skin – and then there was the acne… Not a spot, here and there. Raging acne (probably caused by endometriosis and incredibly bad periods with neuralgic migraines), which had me hiding behind a fringe, unable to look anyone in the eye, trying to disguise myself with too-pink concealer, black mascara and cheap blue eyeliner. In later life I've suffered from an aggressive type of arthritis, viral thyroiditis, psoriasis and other problems which have meant that I've had to fight to maintain the condition of my nails, hair and skin – but I'm lucky, actually, because this has given me such an insight into other people's skin, hair and body challenges. In some ways, having spots and being flat-chested was character-building – but it's horrible at the time, and I empathise hugely with anyone who has visible skin problems, or scarring, or who loses their hair or brows or one of countless other scenarios that impact on their appearance.

I'm dyslexic, so school was no breeze, either – and I got bullied. After A Levels, I wanted to become a beauty therapist. When I told my teachers my plans they looked down their noses at me – but I couldn't see the point of university, because I couldn't see what career path it would lead to. So I did an HND in Beauty at Chichester College (the equivalent of a Diploma of Higher Education today) and haven't stopped learning since. I've studied aromatherapy, reflexology, advanced facials and make-up training, along with more than 20 face and body techniques. I never want to stop learning – and sharing that knowledge. Amazingly, though, even now I get parents telling me they don't want their sons or daughters going into beauty – and I challenge them: why not? It's a multi-billion-pound industry. There are huge opportunities to travel around the world, to make people feel better about themselves all day long – and maybe, one day, even start their own business or found a brand.

My first job was in a hair salon that hadn't previously offered beauty treatments. I had a little room in the back and I'd pay for packets of biscuits, make cups of tea and coffee and ingratiate myself with clients of the Hair Director, Frankie, (who is still my best friend and hairdresser), persuading them to book in with me. I moved on to Grayshott Health Spa in Surrey, working my way up to Head Therapist with a team of 60 and doing treatments on royalty, on household names and on celebrities who'd retreated there to recover from a facelift in seclusion. (And let me tell you: I saw up-close a lot of cosmetic surgery, good and often bad, which has shaped my opinions about why I never want to have this done myself.) I was on first-name terms with supermodels and royalty, but I treated absolutely everyone the same, whether they had a title or were there because their family had saved to send them as a treat after a bereavement or for a birthday day out.

The next step came when I was headhunted by a famous figure in the industry, Clarins's Sales Director Lesley Balls – one of my mentors – who asked me to set up her promotion team and launch Clarins on the first 'A-site' in Selfridges, which is the best spot in the store for grabbing customers' attention. I was responsible for training 4,000 people a year, wrote 22 training courses, designed all their treatments and ping-ponged across the country from Cardiff to Aberdeen, Newcastle to Guildford. I come from the North myself – my strong Geordie accent still comes out when I get a bit heated – and I know very well that not everyone lives in a 'London bubble', and that real people around the country (and indeed, around the world) have many different beauty priorities, needs and budgets. I often went to Paris and spent time in the labs, so I've seen the inside and out of a brand: a 360-degree viewpoint on the industry, which gives me valuable insights.

When I started working for myself, my early clients included ESPA (I set up their training and treatments), Lancôme, L'Oréal Prestige & Collections, Aveda, L'Occitane and many others. I certainly never expected to be on TV, but I was invited to propose some beauty ideas to Peter Ridsdale, then Chief Executive of QVC, the first UK shopping channel, launched in 1993. He planned to launch with some made-for-TV brands that weren't available anywhere else. I told him that, at that time, most people shopped via department stores and high street stores (this was long before the SpaceNKs of this world, let alone websites and social media). I explained that there was a host of fantastic problem-solving brands in salons that weren't on the radar of most beauty shoppers. He liked the idea of showcasing these brands on the channel – I then had the challenge of persuading the brands to get on board, offering the required 30-day money back guarantee. It worked. By Christmas that year, I found myself in front of the camera, and the rest is history.

Through my management consultancy business today, I continue to consult with brands, meeting founders, travelling to labs, helping to develop products, launch strategies and developing training and treatment procedures. But even though I'm a 'beauty insider', privileged enough to be sent new products to try, I still shop like everyone else. I have a dedicated beauty room in my house where I try new products and if I'm walking through Duty Free or a store on Oxford Street, I often splash out on new stuff. It's research, 'test-shopping' to a certain extent. But the bottom line is that it makes me feel as good as everyone else to find a great new cream or feel the mood-boost of a new lipstick or an old favourite. Even to this day, if I'm feeling out of sorts, I will spend an hour locked in my bathroom, washing my hair, using every product and potion at my fingertips, pressing the restart button – and I'll come out a happier person.

We live in an age where people think they're somehow meant to be flawless. Well, we're not. To me, everyone is beautiful. It's too easy right now to feel that you don't measure up to an identikit style of beauty being promoted on Instagram or TikTok, and my aim is to help everyone feel good about themselves, whatever their age, shape, abilities, ethnicity, race, gender or sexuality. I hope every one of you will find something useful in this book, but I acknowledge there is so much more we can do to celebrate all kinds of diversity – because it's those differences that make people beautiful. I welcome the long-overdue steps the industry is now taking to offer make-up for more skin tones and hair types.

Beauty is meant to be motivational; it's not meant to frighten you into buying things you don't need.

Beauty is meant to be motivational; it's not meant to frighten you into buying things you don't need. I long to see everyone walking around with their head held high, feeling good about themselves, without a sense they have to live up to an airbrushed, contoured, filtered, 'perfect' (and also completely unrealistic) cookie-cutter social media or celebrity definition of beauty. (Always remember, these people often have professional help, in their beauty regime and every other aspect of their lives!) Where's the beauty in trying to turn everyone into Thunderbirds puppets or Stepford Wives? (Can you tell I feel strongly about this yet...?) I've never had any cosmetic medical intervention (I'll happily swear an affidavit to that effect!). All my clients' and my own results are from beauty products and my know-how and techniques. There's so much that you can achieve without ever going near a syringe or a scalpel.

This book is my next step on my life-long journey of helping YOU. In the following pages my aim is to cut through the huge amount of confusion about products, techniques, about what you do and don't need. People have become baffled by scientific speak and overwhelmed by the relentless pace of launches – a new *Centella asiatica* cream here, a hyaluronic mask there. In the pages of *The Beauty Insider*, I cover everything from top-to-toe and inside-out: from how to dial up or dial down your skincare routine to make it work for you, to finding the right products to make your hair healthier and shinier, tips that make your make-up stay put longer, how to have sandal-worthy feet, deal with razor burn, or calm your skin by calming your mind. I haven't named specific products, because I'm not trying to sell anything or recommend a price-point that may not be right for you. Instead, I've focused on techniques, approaches and ingredients, empowering you with knowledge to make the most out of your routine and shop the best products in your budget. And throughout, you'll find 'Ask Alison' sections, where I give answers to the problems that I hear time and time again – qualified advice I'd give to a friend or a client. Just a quick warning before we start: always do a patch test when trying a new product, to help avoid any nasty reactions (see p.253).

I've written this book with the idea that it will be a timeless reference book, for beauty customers and professionals too – and I hope it's one you'll leave lying around where you can easily access it, or keep by your bedside. Of course you can read it from start to finish in one session (I'd love that!), but it's written with the idea that it becomes a go-to for you to dip into it whenever you come up against a beauty or grooming challenge, or a friend or family member does. I hope you'll revisit it at different times and stages of life, as your skin, hair and body evolve.

My job – when I bump into you when I'm filling up my petrol tank, on a ski lift or through the pages of this book – is to help you at every step of the way.

Tell me what's great about you!

I really mean that. We need to get much better at being kind to ourselves and acknowledging our good points – and those of the people around us – rather than putting ourselves down.

It isn't surprising that there's a lack-of-confidence epidemic. The beauty industry conspires to make people feel more vulnerable. First up, there's airbrushed advertising imagery. Celebrities who've spent thousands on fillers, Botox and surgery. Or that 'influencer' who's being paid to promote a product (though he or she may have never used it), and then used a filter to make him or herself flawless.

Beyond that, there's the high-tech skin analysis machinery on skincare counters to scare customers into spending money on expensive

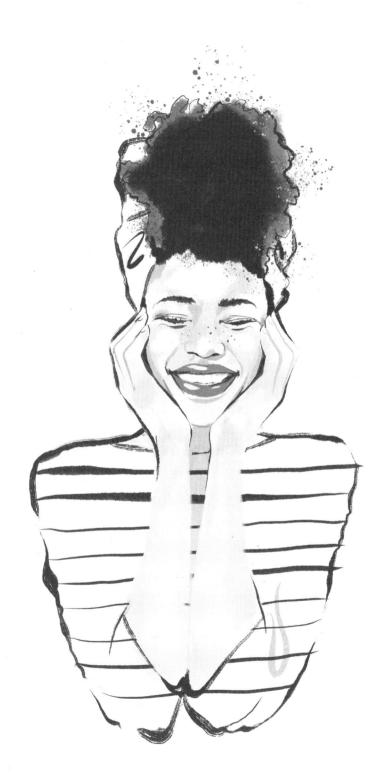

products, using cameras to show them super-close-up imagery of skin on a screen – but never telling you how that compares with others of your age. (And every wrinkle looks like the Grand Canyon up close – even if it's imperceptible to the naked eye in real life. It's no wonder people reach for the credit card at that point…)

The increasing focus on high-tech gadgetry takes all the empathy and communication that the beauty world has prided itself on for so many decades, out of the equation. If you want the black-and-white truth about the condition of your skin, because you've got a major problem, it's always better (if you can afford it) to visit an experienced beauty therapist.

These are just some of the reasons so many people I meet lack confidence about themselves. When strangers come up to me to talk about beauty, often the first thing they'll talk about is something they see as a 'flaw'. I can put my hand on my heart and say I've almost never noticed whatever it is that's bothering them, until they point it out. (And even then, sometimes, only by squinting!) Other people look at the 'big picture' of you – and the age spot that seems the size of Iceland to you is invisible to others.

It's incredibly easy to focus on our 'bad' bits, not our good points. And that's the mindset I want to change, with this book. Positivity really ought to begin in all schools. We should be taught to celebrate our differences, our own individuality, diversity, ethnicity, features, scars, hair. Everyone is different and everyone is important. And on that note, the biggest gift a parent can give their child is to tell them they're gorgeous, all the time, and never, ever to criticise anything about their appearance. Thankfully, schools are starting to have teaching sessions that cover diversity, mindfulness, stress and much more than just spelling and maths. The child who grows up with positive messages will have a sense of confidence that carries them through life.

I believe everyone has an innate beauty. But the reality is our bodies and faces change with the passing of time. When we're growing up, we tend to think that ageing means developing a few lines and wrinkles. We don't realise that all sorts of shifts are going to take place: loss of firmness, change of body shape, a 'fading' of skin tone and hair colour. It doesn't always happen gradually; just as children have growth spurts, we have ageing spurts, perhaps linked to illness, menopause, bereavement. And it certainly doesn't always happen immediately: I'll see people tanning their faces in the midday sun, on holiday, and they'll get away with it for 10 years and then wake up to find lines and pigmentation (because sun damage has a delay factor). We can't stop the clock, so one of the best ways to feel better about ourselves is to stop comparing ourselves with other people. You're you. Uniquely you. That's fantastic!

Let's look at some ways to feel better, right now!

- Give yourself some TLC, in the form of time. A few minutes just to relax and do something for yourself: three minutes to breathe deeply, five minutes to meditate, an hour in the bathroom or having a facial. I absolutely promise you will feel better about yourself (and the world) afterwards.

- Instead of looking in the mirror and thinking, 'I look rough, look at those dark circles,' try to see beyond that so you go: 'Well, that lipstick colour looks great on me. Oh, I'm glad I blow-dried my hair because that really works.'

- When someone compliments you, I'd like you to accept gracefully. We have a tendency, when someone says 'That's a lovely dress?', to say, 'This old thing?' – and to deflect compliments. Instead, smile and say 'Thank you'.

- Start to compliment others, as you go through life. If I'm out and about, I'll often comment to perfect strangers: 'Your lipstick is AMAZING.' Or: 'Your hair looks fab.' Or: 'WHAT a great outfit.' I promise it makes other people feel better, puts a little spring in their step and sends them on their way with an atom more confidence.

Everyone is different and everyone is important.

LET'S WRITE DOWN THE POSITIVES!

I always say to people that for every critical thing you think about yourself, you need to identify three things to compliment yourself on. If you can't think of those, ask a friend or a family member. What I'd like you to do now is take a few minutes to write down all the things about yourself that you like and feel proud of. Shiny hair. Long lashes. Slim wrists or ankles. Deep, velvety brown eyes. Good friends. That you're honest and hard-working (because this is about more than looks). Literally, what's great about you. Try to focus on this list whenever you can, and keep adding to it!

....

....

....

....

....

....

....

....

I'm going to share lots of insider advice over the coming chapters about how you can make the most of yourself, via your skincare regime, your hairstyle, where you apply your blusher (which needs to change every 5–10 years, because our faces change shape!) But at the end of the day, we need to celebrate every line, every scar. Each one is a life experience that's etched itself onto our face or body. A client told me she has a wrinkle for every grandchild – and isn't that a much better way of looking at things, wearing them proudly?

IS THIS ABOUT YOUR DRY SKIN – OR YOUR DIVORCE?

With my experience of treating thousands of clients, I often catch in someone's face and hear in their voice (or read between the lines of a social media post), that while they're talking about something that's troubling them on the surface, it's really all about a deeper life challenge. So: dry skin could be because you don't use the correct moisturiser. But it could *also* be a change of medication, a thyroid imbalance, a recent personal trauma, stress, or the change of the season, to name but a few reasons. We need to look at the whole picture.

Or someone will be talking to me about age spots, but I hear something in their voice, see it on their face, and understand: actually, they're going through a divorce. Maybe a loved one just died. Or they lost their job. Or their kids have flown the nest and suddenly they feel adrift. All of those things can have a massive impact on confidence. So while giving yourself TLC and sorting out the surface stuff is going to make you feel better, seek out help and support for the big stuff and for dealing with life changes. Because mental wellbeing most definitely isn't just skin-deep.

Insider secrets of the beauty industry

I love the beauty industry. The right beauty products and treatments can boost our self-esteem, making us look – and very importantly feel – better. But as a beauty insider, I don't take anything at face value. So here's the truth about the beauty world – and how you can navigate it...

The biggest poblem with the beauty industry right now is the sheer pace of new product launches – it can make us feel overwhelmed and confused. Brands which begin small, promising they'll never launch an eye cream because their one-size-suits-all moisturiser multi-tasks at everything, are pressured by retailers, press and awards to keep up the same relentless pace of launches as the rest of the industry, or risk falling behind. In order to get written up in magazines and newspapers, they also need to offer 'newness' – and so their ranges grow and grow and grow.

Sometimes, after a few years of growing their businesses, those beauty brands will then be sold on to a big company. I don't blame anyone for that. Those founders – so many of whom I've met through my work – work around the clock to become successful. They almost invariably begin in a small room in their home, and spend months if not years tripping over cardboard boxes in the hall as they fulfil orders.

There comes a time, though, that to get to the next level in the beauty world, a successful brand has to take investment – which sometimes means selling the company. Often, they'll stay as spokesperson. And very often, there will be absolutely no difference to you in the quality of their creations, or the values of that brand. Big companies don't buy small brands in order to change them; they tend to buy them because they're doing something they haven't managed to do themselves – reach a particular audience, formulate in a 'cleaner, greener' way, be savvy about social media and build a huge following, whatever.

Customers sometimes tell me that they're disappointed to find that their favourite started-on-the-kitchen-table brand has been 'gobbled up' by a global name, but in most cases, customers will never notice the difference. They won't realise that Liz Earle was bought by Avon and then sold to Boots or that Estée Lauder own M.A.C. and Bobbi Brown, as well as Aveda and Darphin and countless others. Or that Decléor is owned by L'Oréal, and Elemis by L'Occitane. Big companies may well own many different brands, priced from expensive to cheap and the ownership of brands changes constantly because they've become a commodity. The bottom line is that we should be grateful, because the investment that those deep-pocketed companies put into smaller brands, once they've acquired them, powers those small companies to innovate in exciting ways that we can all benefit from. But the fact is no one brand can be great at everything. Just because you loved a brand's first five launches, you can still be disappointed by something they unveil later along the line.

I spend a lot of time investigating ingredients and beauty 'breakthroughs', and I also devote time to researching beauty brands, to discover their ethos and find out about their founders and stories. And that's something I really recommend you do, too; you're putting your skin, hair and face (and your hard-earned cash!) in the hands of these companies. So here are some things to bear in mind, when deciding where to spend yours...

- **Don't automatically fall for skincare fashions.**
There are now fashions in ingredients and products, and I'm not a fan of that. Everything from sheet masks to Amazonian oils via click pens or CICA products are touted as the latest 'must-haves'. Brands scramble to make sure they've got a product in that category too, and we get yet more products. Sometimes, ingredients which have been around for years are given a fancy new name, remarketed, and everyone is suddenly convinced they're the best thing ever! Don't buy something just because there's a buzz about it. Do your own research before believing the hype.

- **Check out/revisit the classics.**

If you find you're baffled by what's happening in beauty and spending money right, left and centre in response to advertising or social media, just pause. I very often point people in the direction of beauty classics: 'heritage' products which have stood the test of time. When you're shopping, always ask which are the top sellers, or the products which have won awards, or have been around the longest. If a product has been on the market for years, that means that customers have returned to it and repeat-purchased because it works.

- **Don't constantly chop and change.**

One of the laments I hear most often is that 'nothing works'. What often happens is that in the quest for the next best thing, we buy products, use them for a short time, and then move on to the next thing – sometimes as soon as the next week. Many products do deliver instant cosmetic benefits such as enhanced radiance or smoother skin, but for significant improvements you might need one, two or three skin cycles (of roughly 28 days each, depending on your age). Read the little instruction books inside before you throw away the box, to see if there are any specific application techniques that can optimise the action of your product. Be patient. Give a product time to work.

- **Don't be 'influenced'.**

One of the trends in the past few years has been the rise of the social media 'influencer', often a young woman paid very handsomely by brands to shoot gorgeous photos of herself using or just holding a product. And that's it. Not really to talk about it, or share knowledge, or even try the product, but just to look good. Influencers are meant to put the hashtag #ad in their comment, but do they always…? Hmmmm.

I find it deeply worrying that an influencer, with no knowledge and no care for the consumers (who often they have never worked with directly), gets X amount of hits and drives X amount of purchases, yet the very next day they'll be pushing something else. I have it written into my TV contract that I don't have to talk about anything on screen that I don't believe in. I only ever recommend brands and products based entirely on my own years of experience and knowledge. I'm also credited with the 'anti-sell', where I'll honestly tell customers NOT to buy something if I don't think it's suitable for their particular skin type or problem!

Seek out authority. Listen to people who've written books or had long-standing columns in the media, who really know their stuff inside out. Be aware, though, that some magazine writers will be encouraged to mention a product to keep an important advertiser happy…

Check out beauty websites and YouTube channels created by truly knowledgeable experts. But to buy a product simply on the strength of a pretty woman or a good-looking boy in a dreamy picture…? Next time you're about to click 'buy', walk around the block. Think about it. Breathe. And you may well find you've changed your mind.

• Models don't really look like that.
On TV, in magazines, on Insta, photos of models are filtered and PhotoShopped and shot from their best angle. They may have had work done too (see p. 144). And although things are improving slowly, only a handful of brands use 'real' women in their advertising.

• Check the small print in advertising.
The trials delivering '100% reduction in wrinkles' or '30% more volume' must be listed in teeny print; sometimes, as few as 20 testers may have taken part. Mascara ads can be especially misleading, meanwhile: those 'false lash effect' mascaras really are often shot on models wearing actual false lashes! By the time the brand is taken to task legally and had its knuckles rapped with a fine for misleading readers/viewers, the mascara's so successful globally that it's a small price to pay for the brand.

- **My advice is: read customer reviews.**

There is nothing like hearing the thoughts of other real people who've tried a product. Many websites now allow customer reviews, and you can be pretty sure if a product you're interested in has had hundreds of five-star or four-star raves, it's good stuff; those comments can also tell you more than the brand's info does about whether it might suit your particular skin type or hair type. (Five stars but only three reviews? Not so impressive. Look for the high numbers.)

- **Look for awards logos.**

Often you'll see that a product has scooped several awards; small brands, in particular, know that winning an industry or media award can really help them stand out in a crowded market. Whether judged by real consumers or industry experts, a winner's logo (e.g. the CEW Awards, the Beauty Bible Awards etc.) is useful signposting to effective products that are worth the money.

- **Research the company behind the product.**

Do you like to support brands that are small and artisan, still run by founder-owners? Or do you like scientifically driven products, which may come from larger brands that can afford to spend millions a year on research and development? Do you want to know about the sorts of charities a brand supports, from saving rainforests to breast cancer research, to see if their values match yours? My advice is to check out the 'About Us' section on any brand's website. You may be able to watch videos of the founder, or the company's most senior trainer or make-up artist.

The bottom line is that we all love and get excited by buying beauty and grooming products, though. We don't always do it because we need something or are looking for a particular result; we can do it – rather like buying a new outfit or a pair of shoes – as a mood-booster. And that's just fine. But by putting yourself in the driving seat to become a more informed shopper, you're likely to make fewer mistakes and waste less money. And who doesn't want that?

How to shop (and not drop!)

We can now shop 24/7 for beauty and grooming products. Here's how to get the best experience, whether you're cruising the beauty aisles or relaxing in your favourite chair...

SELF-SELECTION

There are lots of different retail environments where you pick things off the shelf by yourself: chemists, natural food stores, supermarkets, department stores, etc. In a self-selection setting, there may not be tester units that allow you to sample shades or products for hygiene reasons, so it can be tricky to make the right decision for you. Here are some tips to help:

- **Do your homework before you go.**
  Ideally, go with a shopping list of products/ingredients that you're either replenishing, or which you've researched online before you go, via reviews. You can do this in the shop, through your phone, if you need to do it on the hoof.

- **Be aware of tricks that shops use to seduce you.**
  The expensive products will always be at eye level. More affordable options will be down by your ankles where you really have to look for them – and there really are some fantastic buys at mass-market level. Skincare technologies trickle down from pricy products to the mainstream faster than ever, and mass-market brands like No7, Maybelline, L'Oréal, Rimmel offer amazing value. Some supermarket own-brands have excellent products, too.

- **A bargain's only a bargain if you're going to use it.**
  Self-selection stores often run Buy One, Get One Free (BOGOF) or three-for-two promotions; they're a great way to replenish supplies of something you love, but if you haven't tried a product it's riskier

and you may just end up with three of something sitting in the corner of your bathroom cabinet, unloved.

- **Natural food stores are great sources of info.**
Natural food stores can be a great resource if you want clean/ green/vegan beauty products. The beauty shelves probably won't be officially staffed, but there'll often be sales assistants around, because their customers tend to ask lots of questions about allergies and cosmetics sensitivities, so they're generally very good at steering you towards what you're looking for and answering queries.

Alison's Tip —————————————————————

If you're trying to match a make-up shade, always take your product/s with you. It's impossible to match just from memory.

DEPARTMENT STORE BEAUTY COUNTERS/ BEAUTY STORES

These are stores that offer customer guidance. Whether you shop at a department store or a specialist 'beautique', use your inner compass: seek out a consultant who you think will understand the needs at your stage of life. If you're young and experimenting with make-up, you don't want advice from someone who looks like your mum. If you're a more mature customer, you probably don't want to hear about anti-ageing from someone whose only wrinkles are in her skirt. If you find a sales consultant you really get on with and whose advice you cherish, they'll take good care of you, by being generous with samples or sending you invitations to preview new products. Here are some more tips to make the most of your experience:

- **Again, do your homework before you go.**

As well as looking at brands' websites, check out their social platforms, which give you an idea of their image, target age range, and whether they may have the sort of skin solutions you're looking for. This can be a really useful shortcut to the counters and brands that might be best for you, because walking into any large store puts you on sensory overload, making these spaces hard to navigate successfully. Bear in mind the brands with a wider range of products are more likely to offer more specific options and answers.

- **Large stores have consultants who are paid by one brand.**

They will only give advice and recommend products within that one brand, but they're often incredibly passionate, very highly trained and have given their lives to beauty. The top consultants will have received awards, be incredibly proud of what they do and inspire and train the teams they work alongside. It's a job I've done myself and hugely enjoyed. But you're still only as good as the products themselves, so do research before you go.

- **Specialist beauty retailers (such as SpaceNK, or the beauty hall at M&S in the UK) have consultants trained across a range of brands.**

They're able to offer more independent advice, across a range of brands. You can pick up tips and receive personal recommendations that you just don't get while self-selecting beauty. However, these stores may not stock the whole range of each brand.

- **Be clear about what you're looking for.**

If you want an entirely new cleanser, for example, you'd probably be better served by going to the counter of a big brand that maybe has five or six in their range, rather than a small brand with a slimmer selection. In some cases, you can try-before-you-buy in store via mini-treatments offered in rooms, generally just off the main sales floor. It's always worth asking for samples to try at home, although these may be restricted to newly launched products.

- **Don't be blinded by science.**

Quite often, consultants will use baffling science-speak that they've absorbed in training and big up 'new' wonder ingredients. Do feel free to ask them what it will do for you, and your complexion, or how it will answer your beauty needs.

- **'GWPs' can be excellent for picking up trial sizes of products.**

That's industry-speak for Gift With Purchase; they're fantastic for trying out a dinky size of a cream before swinging for a big size, or for experimenting with a new lipstick shade in a mini. Christmas gift coffrets, often with a selection of downsized products inside, can also offer a great opportunity for trying before you buy. But be aware: the actual bag or box that your gift comes inside may not be made to the same standard as the brand's own products.

BUYING AT SALONS

A facial or a treatment in a salon or spa can be a fantastic way to discover new products, because they're actually used on you in real time. You can decide whether you like the feel, scent, texture, the result – or conversely, if it makes your skin prickle or itch. Lots of us choose treatment destinations because we know and love the range/ranges used, but salons and spas can also be a great way to check out an entirely new-to-you range, up close. Of course, you don't have to book in for a facial or a treatment to shop in a salon for your skincare; you can use them like any other retailer, popping in to buy in person rather than online. It's worth knowing, though, that you can still always ask to speak to a qualified therapist for one-on-one advice.

- **Get the most from your treatment appointment.**

Did you know that you can ring up and request to book the most senior person on the team? Or ask if there's an award-winning therapist on the team? That's often a smart thing to do if you're looking for really good skincare wisdom. It's really helpful to share in advance what you hope to get out of a session so they can do their prep: are you looking for help with a specific beauty problem? They'll be examining your skin with no make-up on it through a magnifying glass in strong light, so they're brilliantly placed to give you answers. Alternatively, you may just be looking for a relaxing, therapeutic experience – in which case, let them know that, too.

- **Only buy what you need/can afford.**
Salons and spas have a tendency to present you with a prescription at the end of the treatment of up to a dozen products used in your session, which are supposedly right for your skin type/challenges. You're in the driving seat, here – don't feel pressured to buy a single one, if you don't want to. But if you would like to buy something, and you're not sure which to splash out on, ask the question: 'If you were me, which would make the most difference to my skin...?'

You're in the driving seat here – don't feel pressured to buy.

ONLINE SHOPPING

There's a wealth of information online about brands and products and this is a fantastic way to research in depth. You can generally find a full ingredients listing, which is good if you know you're sensitive to something, and there are often demo videos. Shopping online is obviously great for accessibility, too. One last bonus: when you shop online, you have almost every product on the market at your fingertips – no matter where you live.

CAN YOU RETURN PRODUCTS?

Cosmetic purchases are covered by the Consumer Rights Act 2015. If you change your mind about a purchase and the packaging is unopened and undamaged, you have 14 days to return it. If products are faulty, you have a legal right to a refund if you return within 30 days of purchase/receiving it, regardless of what the retailer's returns policy is (you can find that on their website and in store). So if something breaks within 30 days (say, a pump on a body lotion, or the hinge on a compact), you're certainly entitled to your money back.

If you develop a reaction to a product, you may well find that the retailer or brand offers a refund, even though they're not legally bound to do so. If you've simply changed your mind, though, you can't really expect a refund. If you don't get anywhere with the sales consultant when trying to make a return and you feel you have a case for getting your money back, you may need to speak to a manager or go direct to the brand's head office.

TV shopping has different rules, often with a 60-day money-back guarantee, so you have two complete skin cycles to see if a cream is right for you, or whether that shampoo really does deliver the ton of volume you were promised.

- **Buy from reputable sites.**

We all want a bargain, but if you go for the cheapest you can find, it may have come via the 'grey' market (a term used to describe unauthorised distributors). The product *may* be fake or copycat, or may be damaged or approaching its sell-by date. There's a wealth of well-known, high-quality online sites, as well as brands' own sites – they all sell direct now. Stick with those.

- **Take advantage of Live Chat, virtual appointments and virtual 'try on' technology.**

Got a question? Often you can have an exchange with someone who can point you in the right direction, if you need more information. Many brands now also offer online tools that allow you to upload a photo to 'try on' a product.

- **Look out for 'Zoom parties' or live events.**

Many brands are now holding events online that give you the opportunity to hear directly from the experts.

Alison's Tip

Be careful when clicking on an advert on Instagram or Facebook. Check before you buy that the retailer is the one you expect, and always check the shipping charges before the final 'click', as these can be incredibly steep. Take a note of what you've ordered and a screenshot of the transaction, to follow up. It's not uncommon for social media purchases not to arrive at all – and it's easy to forget what you've ordered in a busy life.

RELATIONSHIP SHOPPING

Many brands now have representatives who'll come to your house (the most famous being Avon) to show you products and take orders for make-up, skincare, haircare, bodycare and even fragrance. This can be a fantastic way to explore products in a relaxed way – on your own, or with a bunch of friends – with a trained person on hand to offer advice. Just like finding a great consultant in a department store, they can become a go-to for trusted advice and news of launches. But it's important before the first visit to find out what you're committing to: a certain spend, a particular frequency of purchasing, and what the returns policy is if you don't get on with something.

TV SHOPPING

There are now many shopping channels that showcase beauty. One of the huge advantages is there is generally a no-questions-asked money-back guarantee for anything you've bought – as much as 60 days (check the channel's terms).

Of course you would expect me to say this, wouldn't you? But this is why I went to work on QVC in the beginning, because I loved this new approach to selling beauty by educating the customer. (As I mentioned earlier, I have it written into my contract that I don't have to sell anything I don't believe in.) QVC is still one of the longest-standing clients of my beauty consultancy and broadcasting business.

- **These beauty shows are very educational.**
  You get to watch the brand founder, the company's most experienced trainer or the scientist sharing a huge amount of knowledge as they explain the products in depth – basically, you get to hear from the oracle. They may demo a product on a model, and you'll get a real feel for how a product performs. It can arm you with the knowledge and confidence to shop those products, wherever you want to buy them. You can sometimes ask questions through social media that will be answered on air, or you can contact that person direct via their social media after the show is over; if they're doing their job well, you may get a personal reply.

- **You can get some great deals.**
  As with any large retailer, TV shopping channels buy in huge volumes and can pass those discounts on. There can be great

'bundles' on offer – but remember: a bundle is only a bargain if it's something you are going to use. It's a good way to stock up on favourites or share with friends who are fans of that product.

- **You can multitask while shopping!**
You can listen and learn, yet be getting on with something entirely different in your life, e.g. giving yourself a facial, putting on a face mask, cooking, doing the ironing or getting on with a hundred and one other tasks! The other advantage? Simply that you're completely in control. You can switch off without having to say, 'I'm sorry, I'm just looking today,' to anyone.

Shop your cabinet

You don't always need to go out and buy a new product. Casting a fresh eye on the skincare you already own and 'upskilling' with some new techniques may be all you need to rev up your regime…

What does your beauty stash look like? Is it perfectly organised, sorted into categories, all checked to make sure it's within date? If so, I respectfully suggest you flick to the next chapter, with my congratulations!

In reality, most of us need to revisit our beauty products every now and then and have a good tidy-up. Sometimes we go out and buy something new simply because we don't know what we've got. So, before you shop, first assess what you've got and perhaps discover hidden treasures…

- **Organise yourself.**
One of my best tricks is to zone your products so that like is always stored with like. It's amazing how, when you take the time to get organised, you'll discover old favourites. So gather and zone your various cleansers in one place; ditto serums, toners, moisturisers and eye products. The best place to store skincare and make-up is

right where you're going to use it; you can use drawers, baskets or other containers to store items out of sight but unless they're close to hand, you'll almost certainly forget to use them.

If you don't have one specific area devoted to skincare in your life, try to create one. You'll find it so much easier to identify any gaps and then shop intentionally, ideally with a list, which in turn saves you impulse buying. It's surprisingly easy to think you need to go out and buy a face wash, while there's a perfectly good one lurking behind a giant bottle of shampoo.

If you do find you've got lots of moisturisers, say, place them around your home where you might remember to slather some on e.g. by your bedside, on your desk, or for a quick skin-quench while you're watching Netflix.

• Reassess your regime at the change of season.
The start of spring, summer, autumn and winter are good points to switch around your skincare. When the central heating goes on, you'll be reaching for richer moisturisers; as soon as spring comes around, a higher SPF is a must. Regroup, and physically move products that are 'out of season' to the back of that zone.

• Look at use-by dates.
You can work out a product's shelf life via a symbol on the packaging – it's a small symbol with an open-lidded product, with a number of months beside it (6 months, 12 months, 24 months). If you like, buy yourself some coloured stickers and write the date you started using the product on that, and stick it on the bottom of the bottle, tube or jar. If you're unsure whether a product's still safe, use your eyes and nose: has it separated/changed colour? Does it smell off, or just different? Send it bin-wards.

• If you can't bear to throw something out, find another use for it.
Traded up to a more powerful anti-ageing cream before you got to the end of your last product? Facial oil too rich for your complexion?

Use it up on your body and hands, which will always be grateful for the extra TLC.

- **Keep products out of sunlight and away from heat.**
A dressing table is lovely, but not if it's in direct sunlight or beside a radiator. You don't have to keep products in the fridge, but you should keep them away from heat sources and direct sunlight.

- **I'm not trying to put you off shopping!**
We all love buying beauty products; with their gorgeous scents and textures, they're a total mood-lift and a treat for the senses. But if things are tight, you can almost always shop your own beauty stash…

WHEN TO SPLURGE

For me, the main principle is: are you getting great results? If it ain't broke, no need to fix it. But if you'd like to see improvements, or your existing products aren't delivering what you'd like, it may be time to invest in better quality. In the case of hair, for example, you can get away for years with a supermarket shampoo and conditioner, but then one day, wake up and realise I need extra help.

For me, splurging is either to deal with a problem, or for sheer pleasure. There's so much enjoyment to be had from beauty; it is one of the very few things that many of us do exclusively for ourselves, so give yourself permission to treat yourself to something lovely. If you treat yourself to a beautiful aromatherapy bath oil that dials down your stress level and helps you sleep, that may, in turn, benefit your skin.

The other reason to splurge, of course, is when you find an upsized version of a favourite product in a limited edition or at a special price. Bigger sizes are better value – provided it's something you do love and use.

Skin

Embrace your skin and treat it kindly

Your skin is the largest organ of the body. It will change throughout your life, governed by hormones and the natural ageing process. Our skin type is almost always determined by genetics – so my advice is to learn to embrace it and treat it as kindly as you possibly can. I can arm you with the skills to manage it so that nobody can guess whether you're oily, combination or dry. (Because very, very few of us are 'normal'!)

For most people, skin progresses through different stages, from oily to combination, combination to normal, normal to dry.* The skin before puberty is generally in perfect balance and only needs the gentlest of care. As hormones kick in, teenagers tend to become oily, with skin gradually calming down by our twenties so that only the central T-zone of the face stays oily.

If we're lucky, we then go through a 'normal' phase *en route* to becoming dry-skinned, which tends to start in our mid-to-late 30s. That can last for a while – or pass in what feels like the blink of an eye, becoming normal-to-dry, and ultimately dry by the time we reach our 40s and 50s. If you have black, brown or naturally tanned skin, and it's oilier, however, the bonus here is that you won't suffer visible signs of ageing, like lines and wrinkles, until much later, if at all.

Alison's Tip ———————————————————

If you have a teen with oily or 'problem' skin in the family, they need so much TLC. Parents should be aware that as puberty starts earlier than ever, children as young as seven, eight or nine can start to have oily skin. Try to teach them from a young age that they need to be kind to their skin, rather than aggressive. Choose products together that will nourish and protect their skin, rather than harsh products. You'll find more about this on page 112.

———————————

* Be aware, that skin type can change with illness or medication and if this happens out of the blue, consult your doctor.

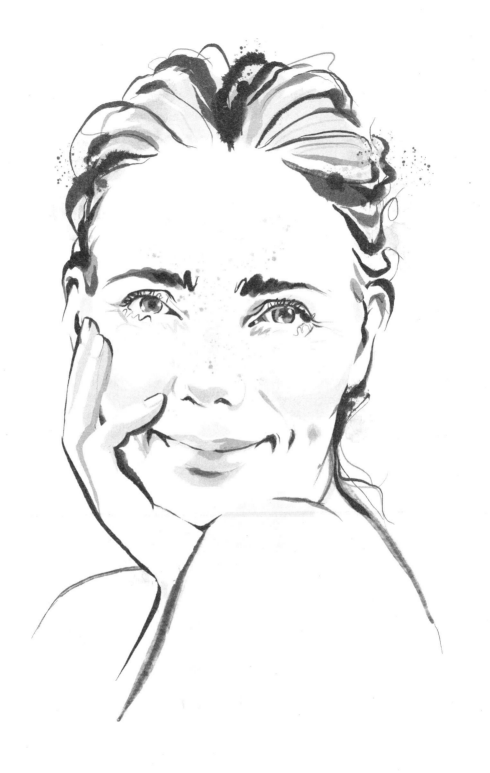

Skin types

OILY SKIN

You have oily skin if…

- your skin is always greasy/shiny.
- your skin never feels dry or tight.
- you have open, often large pores on the face, especially on the T-zone.
- you are prone to blackheads (where plugs of sebum in pores have oxidised).
- make-up (if you wear it) seems to slide off, or shine comes through the make-up.

Traditionally, oily skin is linked with the teenage years. It's a result of the hormonally powered stimulation of the oil/sebum-producing glands at the base of the velus hair follicles (which cover most of the face). Oily skin is also the most blemish-prone – it's not invariably spotty, but for many, the two go hand-in-hand. (See p.108 for dealing with spots/acne.) Men often tend towards oilier skin throughout life in the stubble area and/or the T-zone (see FOR MEN ONLY, p.130).

The natural reaction for most people who have oily skin is to use harsh products in an attempt to banish every last trace of oil. In fact, you need to take a gentle approach, because your skin is overactive. You really do need to 'dial down' what you do to it. You need to avoid harsh, strong products and treatments because they have the opposite effect to what you want, and can make the oil glands produce more oil. I can't emphasise this enough: try gentler products and techniques and you should start to see improvements (also see p.46).

TRACKING IMPROVEMENTS

It can be really helpful to keep a skin diary (maybe with a series of selfies?), to track your skin's progress, as it's very easy to forget how it was last month. You might go down from 17 spots one month to 13 this month, five the next – and it's encouraging to track those improvements. How quickly you see improvements to oily skin depends: men can see results in a month. Women can take up to three months, or three hormonal cycles, to rebalance. Skin tends to be oilier and to break out around periods, so don't despair if you don't see overnight improvements. Judge your skin month by month, not day by day.

DON'T ...

- Use scrubs or masks more than once or twice a month. If your skin is breaking out, avoid scrubs altogether as they shouldn't be used on broken skin.

- Think you can dry out the skin using skin-stripping alcohol-based toners or any other harsh type of product.

- Think you can get away without moisturiser; all skins need moisture and you shouldn't leave skin bare.

- Use cleansing brushes daily, which will over-stimulate the skin.

- Use sunbed treatments, thinking it's going to solve breakouts – it can actually make the oil glands worse by stimulating them.

- Put your face in the sun, no matter what your skin tone; skin will produce more oil as a defence.

- Avoid wearing sunscreen, no matter what your skin tone. Seek out gel-based or spray-based SPFs which are invisible on the skin. Look for the word 'non-comedogenic' on the packaging, which means non-pore-blocking – and always use SPF30, or above.

- 'Dial up' to using stronger products without trying the light approach described below first. (See p.46 for more on this.)

DO ...

- Cleanse with a gentle, non-stripping facial wash in the morning as well as the evening, to remove sebum produced overnight.

- Moisturise morning and night with a lightweight liquid gel or an oil-free moisturiser, including the T-zone. This has the action of calming the skin down.

- Use products with antiseptic and calming ingredients such as tea tree, lavender, chamomile, sage, cypress and/or rosemary, which can help keep skin clean and bacteria-free, but are gentle and soothing, too.

- Remove SPF before reapplying it, if you're spending time in the sun, rather than layering it on. Layers of SPF can trap dirt, grime and sweat, causing pimples. Carry micellar water-soaked cotton pads in your beach bag to clean skin between reapplications.

COMBINATION SKIN

You have combination skin if…

- your T-zone is often shiny (and maybe occasionally spotty), but your cheeks feel tight.
- you have oiliness/breakouts along the jaw-line, and are dry elsewhere (generally an issue with men, or women with a hormonal imbalance, such as endometriosis).
- you can't quite describe what skin type you are as it's different in each area.

Combination skin is confused – and you're probably pretty confused, too, because you're not sure what skin type you have! Sometimes you may think: 'My skin feels normal.' Other times you may think: 'I've got breakouts; it's got much oilier.' This is combination skin: your oil glands are out of balance, which, if you're female is to do with the hormone cycle.

If you're a guy, there can be a contrast between the oily T-zone and the dry beard area (and/or dry cheeks and forehead), but what you have is also combination skin. Conversely, some men can actually have oilier skin along the jawline, dryer elsewhere – but that's still combination.

Many people self-identify as having combination skin, even when most of their skin is normal or dry, with only around 10 per cent of the face prone to shine and oiliness. If you've had oily skin in the past, it can be surprisingly hard to shake off the 'fear of oil', and you'll describe your skin as combination even when it's mostly become normal. This is why you need to assess your skin on a regular basis, to see how it's evolving.

On the skincare 'dial', combination skin is hovering in the middle. If you're too harsh with it, you can dry skin out or tip it further into oiliness. If you don't give it enough moisture, it can become uncomfortably tight. You don't want extremes of ingredients or techniques to overstimulate your complexion – caring for your complexion type is about gentleness and balance, so that you stay in control.

DON'T ...

- Strip skin with harsh products (generally with high levels of alcohol or acids) that leave your skin feeling dry.
- Feel that you need two sets of products for the different areas of your face – tackling combination skin is as much about technique as it is about product, and you don't need to spend a fortune.

DO ...

- Seek to keep skin in balance, as your No.1 priority.
- Use a cleansing milk or wash, rather than the richer types of cleanser such as oils and balms. As your skin gradually rebalances you may be able to move more towards a cleansing balm and gentle, alcohol-free toner.
- Find a moisturising product that is suitable for your whole face – not-too-rich, not-too-light. Apply generously to your drier areas first, and then lightly to oilier areas. Don't be tempted to skip the oily zone, because moisturiser is going to help this area rebalance. You can always double-moisturise thirsty zones.
- Keep the use of scrubs and masks to no more than once every two weeks, or you risk overstimulating your skin.
- Apply lightly antiseptic products to the T-zone if it's prone to spottiness.
- Use eye product and serum when you first see signs of ageing in that area.
- Use a daily SPF, minimum SPF30 for faces, always.
- Try 'multi-masking'; a real trend in recent years, it's fun and effective! Target the oily centre panel of your face with a clay-based mask and a creamy or gel-créme mask where it sometimes feels dry and tight.

Alison's Tip ————————————————————

Be your own skin analyst. We all need to look closely at our skin on a regular basis, to figure out what's normal and when our skin's out of whack. Is it a little dry today, needing a moisture boost in the form of a mask? A little breakout-y, perhaps because it's that time of the month? Are lines and wrinkles stabilising, getting worse or improving?

Every time you get to the end of a product, ask yourself: is this still working for me? It's very easy to be on autopilot with skincare, using the same products month after month, year after year, without really assessing whether they're delivering.

NORMAL SKIN

You have normal skin if...

- you can't really see the pores.
- you don't feel dry, but don't have shine either.
- make-up stays in place well.
- when I ask you: 'What are your skin concerns?', you can't really come up with an answer.

This is the rarest skin type, and if you've got it, you're incredibly lucky! Your skin is more akin to a child's skin, so treasure it. And be aware that it may not last; normal skin is often a phase, *en route* to drier skin as the years roll on. This window often coincides with the highly reproductive years, when the body is in full bloom, including your skin.

Your complexion is in the centre of the dial – neither overactive nor underactive – and it's about preserving that status quo for as long as possible. The good news? You don't need a complicated regime at all.

DON'T ...

- Be scaremongered into thinking you have to buy expensive skincare products or have a complicated regime – a daily cleanse, tone and moisturise, weekly scrub and mask is fine for you.

- Be lulled into thinking that because you've got good skin, you can put your face in the sun. You're not invincible. The damage will always, always catch up with you later, so don't say I didn't warn you!

DO ...

- Choose products on the basis of enjoying them: textures and ingredients you like using.

- Simply use rosewater, if you like, as a great inexpensive toner.

- Try crème-gel products.

- Remember to still use an SPF; this is your most valuable product as it will help maintain your skin.

- Indulge in beauty treatments, both at home and in salons; you can enjoy a DIY facial as often as once a week.

- Add in an eye cream/neck cream if you start to see fine lines or wrinkles; the eye area, upper lip and neck are the first to show signs of ageing.

- Enjoy it. You have the skin equivalent of a unicorn.

Alison's Tip

If you experience a dramatic change in skin type, this can be a medical marker that you need to get checked out. If you suddenly develop raging acne, boils or start sprouting excess hair, or your skin becomes very dry, flaky and uncomfortable for no apparent reason, then you should always get checked out by a doctor.

DRY SKIN

You have dry skin if...

- your complexion often feels tight and uncomfortable, almost as if it's too small for your face.
- you feel like you have to put on moisturiser immediately after you've cleansed.
- you don't have shine or greasiness.
- your face feels like it's 'eating' your make-up, which disappears quickly.
- your pores may be open, but you don't have blackheads or spots (or perhaps only break out very occasionally).
- your skin often looks 'flat'.
- you're drawn to rich, comforting textures, for instant relief.
- skin reacts rapidly to changes in weather or central heating, becoming even drier.

Do you sometimes feel you can virtually *hear* your moisturiser sinking into your skin? Dry skins are thirsty, thirsty, thirsty, especially if they're dehydrated too (see p.45). But the right techniques can keep you comfortable, nourished and plumped up.

Dry skin is caused by the slowing down of your natural oil/sebum production, and lack of NMFs (Natural Moisturising Factors), with the result that your skin doesn't have the lubrication that gives it suppleness and an appearance of radiance. Dry surface cells don't reflect the light in the same way, so skin can look flat and dull. The skin's barrier function becomes compromised, which means that there are literally tiny cracks in the surface which allow moisture to evaporate – it's a vicious circle. A priority is to maintain a healthy barrier through nourishing and protective products, helping to avoid skin becoming sore, red, flaky or rough.

Dry skin tends to be associated with the passing of time – it's what happens as skin's 'metabolism' slows down. You may benefit from rich products that also offer anti-ageing benefits to address slackness or lines and wrinkles, which I talk about more on p.93.

On the skincare dial, your skin is underactive, which means that you need to boost its action. It's higher maintenance than some skin types, but the good news is that with the right techniques and by layering products, you can have the appearance of normal, glowing skin.

DON'T ...

- Go without moisturiser, ever.

- Use harsh toners – only the gentlest products for you.

- Use clay-based masks – they're much too drying.

- Splash out on lots of different moisturisers; just use the ones that you have more lavishly and frequently!

DO ...

- Opt for balm/oil/cream cleansers – anything else is too light for you.

- Use richer products, more often: oils, butters, creams and serums.

- Double-dose – or even triple-dose. This means applying product once, then a second time when it's sunk in. Even a third time, if you're home in the evening. If you get up in the night to go to the loo, slap some moisturiser on then, too!

- Learn to layer products. This is the No.1 secret for dry skin. You may not feel moisturised enough with just a moisturiser; you will if you layer a few drops of facial oil and/or serum underneath. Customise and play around till you reach your perfect comfort level.

- Use masks and exfoliants. These are a dry skin's best friends, because they stimulate your underactive oil glands. Gentle exfoliation also helps to slough off the flat, dead surface cells that make skin look dry. A light scrub or enzyme exfoliant also 'preps' skin for a long drink of moisture in the form of a rich, creamy mask which you may leave on overnight.

- Be sure to use adequate SPF (minimum SPF30, ideally SPF50); dry skins are the most prone to signs of ageing.

- Remember: more is always more, with dry skin.

Skin conditions

As well as understanding your skin type it's important that you understand the symptoms of a couple of common skin 'conditions' that can come and go. These are problematic states for skin that anyone can suffer from, no matter what your skin type. You must treat these conditions first (especially sensitivity) before addressing issues with your skin type or ageing.

SENSITIVITY

People often tell me they have 'sensitive skin,' but this is a real misconception, because sensitive skin is a temporary condition. If you've been experiencing sensitivity for years, you really are using the wrong products, which may be too active, or in some way irritating. Sensitive skin tends to flare up intermittently, and it shows as flakiness, stinging when you apply a product, irritation, itching or raised lumps and bumps under the skin. What's really important is to look at your whole routine and dial it right down, to calm things (see p.46). Find the gentlest cleanser and moisturiser that you own, and just use those for a few weeks. No 'extras': forget about masks, exfoliators, serums and even separate eye products.

Nowadays, skincare ingredients can have 20, 30, 40 or more ingredients listed on the back, and any one of those can be a trigger, so identify the products with the shortest ingredients list, and use those. For moisture and nourishment, try using just a few drops of a single base oil such as rosehip or sweet almond. Wait for your skin to get back into balance, and then one by one, reintroduce products. Leave a few days between each reintroduction and be alert for signs of sensitivity; you might even want to keep a skin diary to track things.

This should help you to narrow down whether it's a particular skincare product triggering the flare-up, such as a supposedly 'gentle' peel that was too active for your complexion.

I've also been caught out in the past by using a favourite product that proudly announced itself as 'New and Improved', but something in that new formulation caused a reaction.

Do be aware, though, that the flare-up could also be triggered by a new washing powder, a room spray, or even a food or a change in medication (also see p.33). It can sometimes take a little detective work before you hit the nail on the head. If you think it's a change in a prescription that might have caused it, seek medical advice.

DEHYDRATION

Dehydration is a condition almost all of us will suffer from at some point (whatever your skin type) and it's more prevalent these days. Skin (indeed the whole of our body) is made up of mostly water – it keeps each cell plump and healthy. Our sweat should mix with our natural sebum to create a perfectly balanced, moisturising surface layer – but this is really only found in babies and toddlers. When our skin becomes dehydrated it loses water content and the cells function less efficiently. Skin can look dull, deflated and ashy, and lines can appear more prevalent. Because our skin is out of balance, sensitivity can occur too.

Even young and healthy skin can get dehydrated with late nights and stress. This can even give you what appears to be wrinkles but are actually fake lines caused by the skin shrivelling. You need to drink more water, get more sleep and apply hydrating products – ideally a serum, gel or moisturiser containing hyaluronic. As you get older, dehydration can be a constant battle and it can be made worse by multiple factors: tiredness, long days, heating, air con, sun, illness, certain skin products and even wearing make-up for long periods. However, it should be easy to solve; add more water-based ingredients to your routine and layer with oil-based ingredients, to trap in hydration. You can also try multi-molecular hyaluronic formulas. Serums, balms, oils and moisturisers can have a dramatic effect quickly, and there's no need to spend too much. You may just need to layer your products (see p.43) or add a hydrating mask to your routine.

Note: if your skin is oily or spotty, but also flaky, it's dehydrated too and it's more likely to scar. Treat dehydration quickly and you'll get a quick result; don't treat it and it can lead to sensitivity or increased ageing in the long term.

How to dial up or down

I talk a lot about 'dialling up' and 'dialling down' because this is a really easy (and often budget-friendly) way to make your skincare routine work better for *you*. Rather than reaching straight for the next trendy product, think about whether your routine is working for you first and whether you need to turn the dial.

Dial up

If your skin is dry, tired or you've started to see signs of ageing, it is underactive and it may need a boost. You can turn up the dial on your routine with stronger ingredients, like peptides, retinols and acids, but there are also several other ways you can do it. You could introduce products with more complex formulas, start a regime of stronger exfoliation or use techniques like massage or electrical therapies to stimulate your skin - and of course you can do each of these things more often, or even just try your usual products and techniques more often.

Turn the dial gradually (don't leap straight to using strong acids if you've never used them before) and beware: stronger ingredients and techniques *can* lead to effects we're not looking for, like sensitivity or spots. If that happens, turn the dial back down...

Dial down

If your skin is sensitive, or overactive and oily, you could benefit from adjusting your routine so that you reduce the stimulation to your skin. Strip back to single-ingredient products, gentle ingredients like plant waters and oils (which have a pH very similar to your skin) and less frequent and less invasive exfoliation and techniques. Once your skin has rebalanced, you may want to introduce stronger ingredients and techniques, but go extremely carefully. A gentle routine may be all you need.

Also see the pH scale on pp.128–29 to understand where key ingredients sit on the scale compared to your skin. Only venture outside your natural pH zone with care.

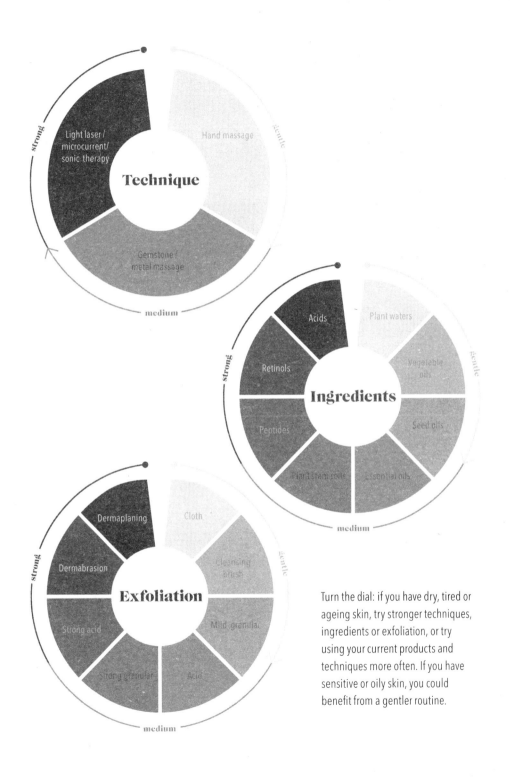

Technique

- Light laser / microcurrent / sonic therapy
- Hand massage
- Gemstone / metal massage
- strong
- gentle
- medium

Ingredients

- Acids
- Plant waters
- Retinols
- Vegetable oils
- Peptides
- Seed oils
- Plant stem cells
- Essential oils
- strong
- gentle
- medium

Exfoliation

- Dermaplaning
- Cloth
- Dermabrasion
- Cleansing brush
- Strong acid
- Mild granular
- Strong granular
- Acid
- strong
- gentle
- medium

Turn the dial: if you have dry, tired or ageing skin, try stronger techniques, ingredients or exfoliation, or try using your current products and techniques more often. If you have sensitive or oily skin, you could benefit from a gentler routine.

FOMO (FEAR OF MISSING OUT)

FOMO is what drives some people to over-complicate their beauty regimes. That, and pressure from social media and advertising, which constantly bombard us with images of people looking young and perfect. There are now 'fashions' in skincare, too, just as there are with clothes and accessories: if we don't have a CICA cream or an azelaic acid serum, we're made to think we're somehow missing out. It's simply not true. (And in reality you've probably used these ingredients before under different names)

Back to basics

Your optimum daily beauty routine doesn't mean a groaning bathroom shelf. Here's the low-down on what everyone 'needs' – and the occasional 'extras' that can make a difference.

Getting 'back to basics' is about personal choice. It's a financial choice and a lifestyle choice, but also dictated in part by how much time you want to devote to your daily regime. The reality is that most of us need fewer products than we've come to believe necessary – so here's what I prescribe for everyone, plus the 'add-ons' that you can turn to for an occasional boost.

THE ESSENTIALS

Choose products that you love using, that you enjoy for their scent or their texture or both. Because when you really look forward to the pleasure of using a product, you'll do so diligently – and that's when you'll see real results. So here's what every skin really needs:

Cleanser

A cleanser does the obvious – it sweeps away the day, taking grime, dead cells and make-up with it. Through the gesture of massaging the skin, it also does the important job of bringing to it oxygen and nutrients. It also prepares the skin for what's coming next. If you don't cleanse properly and thoroughly (and I share how-to techniques on pp.54–55), whatever you put on next won't penetrate in the way it's meant to.

Many brands promote the fact that their cleansers are suitable for all complexions, but if you want to embark on a programme of dealing with a particular skin type – making an oily skin less oily, boosting the moisture in a dry complexion or taking down sensitivity – you may want to start with a skin-specific cleanser. If you use an all-in-one cleanser, occasionally you may need to step up or dial down your routine to manage a particular problem, or add in a specific toner (more about this on pp.46–47).

I advise everyone to cleanse immediately when they get home at night – and the same applies if you're working from home: cleanse in the early evening. There are several good reasons for this:

- If you cleanse when you first come in, you won't be so tired, so you're more likely to do a thorough job than if you're half-asleep just before bedtime.

- The sooner you cleanse your skin when you come in, the more hours you have for the creams and serums you apply to get to work and deliver their skin benefits. I'm a great believer in 'double-application'; if you apply an eye product or a moisturiser when you get home, and it's 'disappeared' by bedtime, you can apply a second time for extra benefits.

- Your cleansing ritual is also an important punctuation mark at the end of the day. It's a moment for mindfulness, a gear-shift, a break from the day. (For more about mindfulness, see p.331).

- It's also about hygiene. Just as you might take off your shoes, rather than bring that dirt inside, think about your face in the same way. You'll be getting rid of pore-blocking make-up, dirt and bacteria, allowing your skin to balance again.

Alison's Tip

Make sure when you cleanse that you can access every bit of your face and neck from hairline to bust-line. Clip or tie your hair off your face so that you can reach the hairline and the ears (and behind the ears). Take off any jewellery and be naked above the chest-line.

Cleansing balms

First popularised by facialist Eve Lom, these are blends of oils, solidified with waxes, which melt and soften on contact with skin. This emulsifies make-up, dirt and debris ready for removal with a muslin cloth or a soft flannel. Cleansing balms are also becoming increasingly popular with male skincare shoppers, I'm finding.

Cleansing creams

These thick, creamy cleansers really do their job best when massaged well into skin, which in turn brings blood flow and oxygen to the face. If you love the texture and/or the scent of your cleansing cream, that's what counts.

Cleansing milks

These are more liquid than creams, akin to a thick milk or runny cream. If you love them, great, but be sure to remove well. A salon technique is to remove with a large tissue, pressed onto the face, so you don't need to use water. (Especially useful if you're sensitive to water, or travelling.) Cotton pads can also be used. Or you may find you get more effective results from switching to a wetted cloth or flannel when you remove the milk.

Cleansing oils

You'll never persuade someone with oily skin to use a cleansing oil if they don't want to, because the texture reminds them of exactly what they're trying to get rid of. For normal to dry types, though, they can be a nourishing choice – they're also really enjoyable to massage into skin, which in turn boosts glow.

My caveat is that although beauty brands often say their cleansing oils (or any all-in-one cleanser) can be used in the eye area, they can trigger sensitivity in some people. If you do use an oil for cleansing the eye, wet a cotton pad first and then add a little of the oil to the pad, rather than massaging the oil directly into the eye zone. Wipe the pad over the eyes, working into lashes, and use a clean pad for each eye. If you find that your eyes become red, sore, irritated or even that a 'film' is left on the eyeball which affects your vision, you 100 per cent need a separate, dedicated eye make-up remover (see p.62).

Face washes

Perhaps unsurprisingly, many have returned to facial washes, a reflection of the world becoming so hygiene-conscious. Google searches for this style of cleanser have been off the scale.

Once upon a time, face washes were the main go-to for people who liked the feel of water on their skin. But now that so many cleansers can be used with water, you have many other options. If you do really like a wash, experiment, because the textures vary wildly; some are richer and creamier, to be worked into skin before adding water (and may be fine for dry skins). The more foaming, sudsy washes will often be too stripping for normal-to-dry or dry skins.

Face washes are ideal choices for men, including anyone with facial hair, as quite high levels of bacteria can lurk in beards and moustaches.

Micellar cleansers

These clear, often fragrance-free liquids work a little like a magnet; they attract particles of dirt via 'micellar technology', a bit like an e-cloth attracts dust. Micellar waters were originally introduced into the beauty world from ophthalmology in Paris, to help women there deal with the region's famously hard water. Used with cotton pads, they'll get your skin clean, but they don't put anything back, unlike creams, oils, balms and milks. They can be used nightly, are great when you're in a hurry, and are perfect as the first step of a 'double cleanse' (which I explain on p.83). You can now also buy micellar oils, which are lightweight cleansing oils that use dirt-attracting micellar technology – and those you CAN use every night.

Cleansing wipes

I don't particularly like cleansing wipes, but they have their place. If you don't have access to water, if you're in hospital or perhaps at a festival, they are better than going to bed with your make-up on. They take quite a bit of friction to remove make-up, and they're not that good at absorbing. That 'drag' isn't good for skin, so keep these for emergencies only. They can also cause sensitivity around the eyes and accelerate ageing. As single-use products, they are also not great for the planet.

Alison's Tip

Never go 'naked'. If you are having a long soak in the bath or shower, leave your cleanser on your skin while you soak or put on a facial oil or mask; it will add a layer of protection. Remove it before you get out of the water, just before you remoisturise. (Don't do this with a face wash, though, as these have detergent elements which shouldn't sit on the skin.)

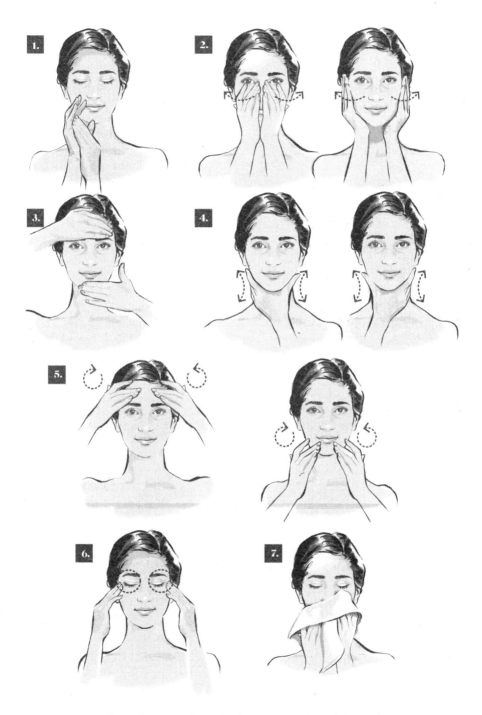

How to cleanse your face with a cleansing cream, lotion, balm or oil

How to cleanse your face

This is the technique for removing dirt and make-up with a cleansing cream, lotion or balm, micellar oil or other cleansing oil. You can complete your nightly cleanse in a minute or two, with the right products, but if you're double-cleansing (see p.83), you'll want to devote a bit longer. Use it as an opportunity for a mindful moment.

1 Massage a generous quantity of your chosen product between your palms; you want the product to remain on the surface of the skin, rather than be absorbed, so you need plenty. Stop to inhale its beautiful smell for a few seconds.

2 Use both hands throughout, mirroring the movements. Avoiding the eyes for now, work the cleanser into your face, using sweeping side-to-side movements.

3 Use outward strokes to sweep the product over the forehead and lower part of the face.

4 Take your cleanser down your neck and massage it into the skin with upward sweeping movements.

5 Use smaller circular movements to remove make up from any congested or lined areas.

6 Last of all, massage around the eyes and eyebrows lightly; if you have slackened skin, support the eye area by placing the opposite hand over your brow to 'tether' it.

7 Soak a flannel or muslin cloth in warm water and use it to gently remove traces of cleanser and make up from the eyes first, using a different, clean piece of cloth for each eye. Cleanse the rest of your face with another clean area of the cloth, working from the centre of your face outwards. Finish by wrapping your cloth around a fingertip and working in small, circular movements into the nose fold and chin. Whatever your skin type, follow with cotton wool pads lightly soaked in toner (see p.56) to remove any last traces of cleanser and dirt.

TONERS

Toners – sometimes also called 'fresheners' – are liquids designed to remove remaining traces of make-up as the final step of your cleanse, before applying serums or moisturiser. And they work: no matter how thoroughly you've cleansed, if you go over the face with a toner you will look at the cotton pad afterwards and see traces of make-up or dirt that were left in your eyebrows, around the hairline, behind the ears or the folds around the nose. If just left there, these can lead to blackheads, breakouts, dryness, flakiness or sensitivity. As far as I'm concerned, toning is still an essential step for all skin types. Choose a simple, alcohol-free toner that will balance the pH of the skin and allow products to sink in better. Floral distillates (rosewater/orange blossom water) are good, too.

Toners are used in professional facials to remove the residues of masks and exfoliants and you're missing a trick if you don't have one in your regime. They're super-versatile; use them before reapplying facial SPF (see p.289), and at the gym or pool to remove any sweat or chlorine.

You could store toner-soaked pads in the fridge in a plastic container for a hot weather cool-down. Would I suggest you keep your bottle of toner itself in the fridge? If you're going to forget about it because it's out of sight, no. However, if you find it refreshing – perhaps you're menopausal, or living in a muggy flat, it can be divine to walk to the fridge and cool your face down with toner.

Some toners are available in mist form – an ideal cool-down at your desk. But for a toner to be truly effective as part of your cleansing routine, it needs to be wiped off your face, bringing the dirt with it, not spritzed and left there. Spritz-on toners are sometimes easier to use on stubble areas, but above the beard-line, toner should still be wiped on using a pad, for best results.

Alison's Tip

I like to leave skin a tiny bit damp from a toner, and then when I apply a cream, serum or an oil, it helps the product to sink in beautifully.

Toner how-to

Brilliant for rebalancing skin's pH after masks, after showering, or at any stage following the removal of products during a facial. And I promise, no matter how carefully you cleanse, there will be traces of it on the pads you use for toning, afterwards. It's essential in hard water areas to rebalance the PH of your skin.

1   Whether you have a 'pouring' toner or a spritz-on, I prefer to apply the product generously to two cotton pads. That gives you four sides to work with.

2   Using two cotton pads at the same time, tucked inside the two middle fingers of each hand, work outwards from the centre of the face.

3   Flip the pads over to the clean side and go down the neck area and behind the ears (you probably have no idea how dirty it gets there!); if you've been using bronzer or make-up down to a v-neckline, sweep all the way down there too.

MOISTURISER

You can't get enough moisturiser. When it comes to moisture, more is more. You don't need an expensive moisturiser; there are some great bargains – it's about finding your favourite texture, and being generous with it.

Moisturiser is for putting back the oil and water that are naturally produced by young skin. Children don't have breakouts and their skin is in perfect balance, actively regenerating all the time, which is why when you look closely, you can't see so much as a pore. But from teenage onwards, that balance is disturbed. This happens at roughly the same time we tend to start wearing make-up, which needs to be removed, also putting skin out of whack. So from teenage onwards, skin needs additional oil and moisture to ensure a healthy hydrolipidic film (hydro = water, lipids = oils). You might sometimes see this called the 'acid mantle'.

People with oily and combination skin sometimes shy away from moisturiser, but every skin, even oily skin, needs moisturiser in the morning and at night, because sebum and oil aren't moisture. Men often shy away from moisturiser, too, and are often blown away by the comfort factor when they finally get round to using one. Whatever your gender, whatever your age, whatever your skin tone or type, moisturiser is a MUST.

Everyone needs to find one moisturiser that is their Little Black Dress of a moisturiser to which they return time and time again. It's your 'base' moisturiser, your great moisturiser love, the one that offers the perfect level of comfort and moisture and can be used morning and night when you want to pare back your routine. It doesn't need to be anti-ageing or have other actions; it just needs to have the correct balance of oil- and water-based ingredients for you and it's just there to make your skin feel great.

Shop according to your household budget. There are creams at 'Mercedes prices', but there are also excellent creams for under £10 – and at every price-point between. In fact, ingredients start out expensive and then 'trickle down' to the mass market at much more affordable prices, so whereas once upon a time if you spent £5 you'd get mostly mineral oil, some parabens and some perfume, it's a very different story now. There are really affordable creams that harness peptide technology or hyaluronic acid (see INGREDIENTS MATTER, p.114). But don't be swayed to buy a product just because it's a 'bargain'. A bundle of three creams at a knock-down price is not a steal if they're not something you already love or are going to use.

Find a product with a texture that you love and which leaves your skin perfectly comfortable. For oily skins there are wonderfully light, almost gel-textured moisturisers, often based around soothing aloe vera. The new cream-gel (crème-gel) textures often appeal to normal/combination skins, and richer creams for dry skins.

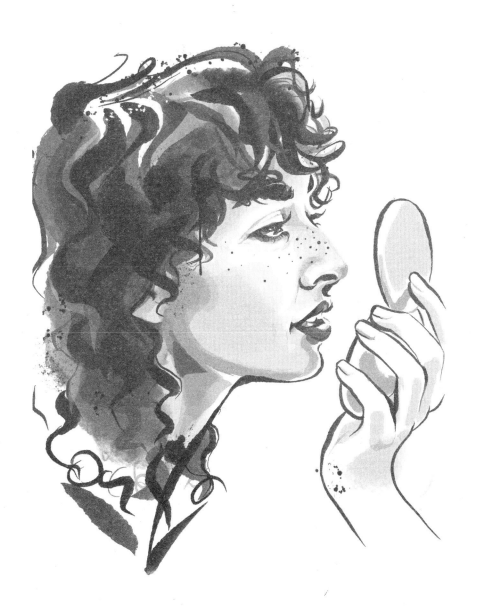

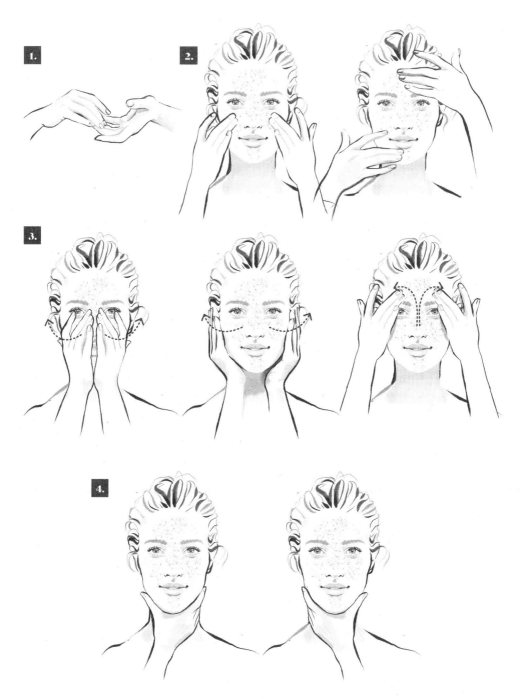

Moisturiser how-to: how and where to apply

Moisturiser how-to

1 Apply your moisturiser using the two middle fingertips of each hand (to save product and money).

2 Press the moisturiser into your skin by placing your hands on the face vertically at the cheek level, then horizontally on your forehead and chin.

3 Mirroring your hands, blend into the skin using fingers outwards and upwards, to get the product into the pores. Be sure to moisturise the centre panel of the face.

4 It is also important to sweep the product down the neck, which is prone to ageing.

DAILY SUN PROTECTION

There's a lot of talk about the need to use a daily moisturiser featuring a built-in SPF. Only an SPF30 or above is adequate for your face, and should be used on any day when you're going to expose your skin to the sun for more than just a few minutes – even if you're just getting from A to B. This means throughout the winter too. It has emerged more recently that SPFs are also good for shielding skin from the blue light emitted by screens, so useful even if staying indoors!

I recommend using a dedicated facial sunscreen OVER your regular moisturiser to ensure adequate protection. The reason for this is that in a daily moisturiser, which is meant to do 'double-duty', some of the goodness or moisture factor in your cream has had to be reduced, to make way for the SPF.

For proper facial sun protection against damaging UV rays, you want the type of sunscreen that is a 'once-a-day' formula, or a specific repeat-application facial SPF that you can regularly top up if sunbathing or for other sun exposure. I'll talk about this layering in more depth in the Golden rules section (see p.284).

THE ADD-ONS

Over and above the basics, there are extras you may want to add in if you wear make-up, or have more mature skin with visible lines, wrinkles or loss of radiance.

Eye make-up remover

If your cleanser doesn't do a thorough job, irritates your eyes or leaves them misty, you definitely need a dedicated eye make-up remover – either a shake-before-use 'dual-phase' remover (the shaking action blends the oil and water layers), or a clear liquid.

Puffy eyes, ageing eyes and slackened eyes all respond to using a separate eye make-up remover. If you have sensitive eyes, these are best for you, too, to keep any oils (which feature in most all-in-one cleansers) away from the eye zone.

Alison's Tip ———————————————————

If you like an intensely pigmented lipstick, an eye make-up remover can be the best way to remove that too!

Eye make-up remover how-to

1   If you're using a separate eye make-up remover, use this before removing the rest of your make-up. Apply the liquid to two cotton pads and hold one over each eye for several seconds to start dissolving the make-up. (You must use a separate pad for each eye to prevent any bacterial cross-contamination.)

2   Place the opposite hand over your brow, to support the eye area from above and stop it being tugged downwards as you work.

3   Sweep one pad over that eye, in a downwards and outwards direction. When that area of the pad gets covered in make-up, flip it over and repeat the downwards and outwards sweeping motion.

4   Fold the cotton pad to create a point which will help you access the lash-line to remove mascara and eyeliner. You can keep folding and creating points, until it's all cleansed.

5   With the other pad (never the same one), repeat on the other eye, swapping the supporting hand.

Eye treatment

You may benefit from an extra eye product to awaken the eye area, even as young as the exam years. Staring at screens, poring over books and staying up late can trigger dark circles and dehydration. Tiny lines and wrinkles may start to show by the end of your twenties. The younger you are, the lighter the texture of eye treatment you should be looking for: a gel or a serum, or a very lightweight cream is ideal, moving up to richer products as the decades go by, when crêpiness, pigmentation and sagging may start to bother you.

The traditional way to apply eye products is to 'tap' them on the brow-bone and upper cheekbone (known as the 'orbital bone'), to minimise the risk of product travelling via fine lines and wrinkles into the eye. But there are now products that can be taken right to the lash-line.

You can step up your regime to see if you can do this with an existing eye product without irritation:

- Apply the eye product more generously than you normally would, as an 'eye mask' treatment. Rest with your eyes closed for 15 minutes before removing.

- If there's a hint of irritation, soreness, redness, or puffiness, do NOT use this product any closer to the eye than that orbital bone, on an ongoing basis.

- If it doesn't cause a problem at all, move on to using it on the lid and closer to the under-eye on a regular basis. Go back to your original 'orbital' technique if at any point you get any irritation or puffiness.

With treatment products, it's a constant process of self-assessment, to see what works, because we're all individuals.

Facial oil

I adore facial oils, and I'm not alone; they're widely loved for their comfort factor and by men in particular for pre- and post-shave use. Although they're an optional 'extra', they have a great affinity with your skin's own chemistry and at some point, you'll benefit from adding one into your regime. Apply them after cleansing and before (or instead of) moisturiser. If you're using a serum, use this before your oil. If you happen to be using all three – serum, facial oil, moisturiser – that's the order to apply them in.

Oils vary, from simple nut and seed oils through to complex blends in which these 'base' oils are infused with active essential oils. If you have sensitive skin, try a base oil of rosehip, camellia or olive, used on its own. If you have drier skin, those oils are also suitable – and so is jojoba oil, which is richer and heavier. Even oily and combination skins can benefit from facial oils, in particular, grapeseed, which has a featherlight texture. (Trust me: it will have a rebalancing action, rather than make skin greasier.) All these base oils can be applied directly to skin.

When you buy branded facial oils, these almost always include a blend of aromatherapy essential oils. These not only smell wonderful; these botanical oils work as 'instructions' to the skin to behave in a particular way – and the labels should tell you which skin types they're suitable for.

There are now some super-high-tech oils with peptides and stem cells, for a turbo-charged anti-ageing action. These targeted treatment oils should be used nightly, but if you're just using them for a nourishing boost rather than a specific 'result', two or three times a week is fine. In this case, it's about finding one that fits the 'pleasure profile', as well as that suits your skin.

What I perhaps like most about facial oils is that they encourage you to massage your face for longer, because it can be such a delight to apply them, and that will show in restored glow.

Facial oil how-to

1 Facial oils are best warmed on the skin by applying a few drops to your palms and massaging them together. (You won't waste product because your palms aren't absorbent.)

2 These blends are often beautifully fragrant, with aromatic essential oils; take a moment to breathe the scent in for a moment of calm.

3 Place your hands together as if you were praying, then separate the hands and smooth in the oil from the nose outwards, mirroring the movements with both hands. Keep the product well away from the eye area.

4 Place one hand horizontally on the forehead, the opposite horizontally on the chin, and continue to massage the face with outward sweeps.

5 Apply the oil down the neck area to the décolletage with further long, smooth strokes.

Alison's Tip ─────────────────────────

If you experience puffiness or 'morning face', that may be down to applying a facial oil too close to the eye area. Imagine a circular 'exclusion zone' taking in your brow-bone to the top of your cheekbone, and keep oils well away from that area.

Serum

if you want skin 'stimulation', to get visible benefits such as brightening, line reduction or pigmentation reduction, a serum can be worth adding into your routine. The water-based composition of serums, which tend, as a result, to be quite light, enables formulators to pack them with scientific ingredients such as vitamins, peptides and high-tech molecules.

Serums can be eye-wateringly expensive – the moment a brand adds an 'anti-ageing' tag to a product, the price can sky-rocket. Never, ever, be persuaded to go beyond your budget for skincare; there really are great products at every price-point.

If you're going to use a serum, this isn't a once-a-week thing. It must become part of your routine in order to see benefits – ideally, both morning and night. A few drops of serum before moisturiser is generally prescribed, but stop this method if you see 'roll-off' effect, whereby the surface of the skin starts pilling. It's not your skin coming off; it's an interaction between products, and it shouldn't happen. If it does, try combining it with a different moisturiser, or choose a serum and moisturiser from the same brand, which will have been tested together to make sure this doesn't happen.

Exfoliators

An exfoliator can help brighten the skin, banishing dullness. This is often especially useful in winter, or after a holiday when your real/*faux* tan is fading and patchy. Exfoliators can also slightly thin the appearance of a wrinkle. There are three types of exfoliator:

- **Physical exfoliators.**

These are the traditional facial scrubs that have been around for years. Jojoba beads are widely used as the exfoliating ingredient in scrubs, but they do absolutely nothing on my skin, skimming over the surface. I prefer a salt or sugar scrub, used only on damp skin. Avoid nut-based scrubs at all costs because these scratch and abrade the skin.

- **Chemical exfoliators.**

These can be enzyme-based (gentler) or acid-based (stronger, for 'resistant' skin). In the form of creams, gels or lotions, massaged into the complexion and left on for the prescribed amount of time before removal, they 'dissolve' the very top layers of skin, revealing new and brighter layers below. Enzyme exfoliators needn't be harsh and in some cases can be kinder to skin than scrubs.

- **Microdermabrasion products.**

These are particularly powerful exfoliators, sometimes based on tiny crystal particles. This type of product was once only available in dermatologists' offices, so proceed carefully: the more powerful the exfoliator, the gentler your technique should be; massage into skin, using your ring fingers to make gentle circles, using the lightest pressure. You can also get microdermabrasion machines, which also use tiny crystals – and the next level up is dermaplaning, a professional treatment that involves gently scraping the skin with a scalpel. (NB These are not suitable for sensitive skins, ever.)

- **Exfoliating brushes.**

Cleansing brushes can have an exfoliating as well as a cleansing action. See p.91 for more about these. Be sure not to use over-zealously.

How often you use an exfoliator boils down to your skin type and its condition: exfoliating is a stimulating procedure so you do it less on oily, problematic skin and more on a dry, ageing, underactive skin. If your skin is **overactive, oily/combination**, I suggest you exfoliate just once a month. You may think a scrub makes your skin feel extra 'clean' if it's oily, but actually what you should aim for is to *rebalance* your skin – which means not overdoing anything. If you are **spotty** or have breakouts, use an exfoliator once a fortnight or a maximum of once a week. Exfoliate right after your period when your skin is calming down naturally.

If you have **dry skin**, two or even three times a week is fine to exfoliate, to keep skin bright by ridding it of flat, dry, dead surface cells.

'Gentle' should be your watchword, always, whatever your skin type. Light pressure, always. This is your precious face – not your floor.

Face masks

When your regular daily skincare isn't delivering quite what you need, reach for a mask. A good mask will, in just a few minutes, deliver real, visible benefits, the kind normal skin treatments would deliver after several days of use. You should be able to look in the mirror afterwards and see a perceptible difference. That might be calmed redness, perhaps, or a skin-quenched plumpness if your skin is dry. Or radiant brightness if you were looking grey and dull. If a mask isn't delivering results you can see, it's not worth what you paid for it – whatever price that was.

Face masks come in all shapes and sizes and at all sorts of price points. But I have to say, I'm often horrified by what is charged for single-use sheet masks, which are basically a bit of paper, with not much product soaked into it. Sheet masks are easy to keep in the fridge, yes. They are great for travelling on an aeroplane or having in your overnight bag, but you'd be much better off getting a 50ml pot of face mask and using that.

If your skin is active (breaking out, oily, spot-prone), use a mask once a month. For combination skin, two or three times a month is ok. For normal, once a week is ok. And if you have dry skin, two or three times a week is ok – you might even sleep in the mask some nights.

Alison's Tip

When I talk about your 'face', am and pm, all products should go down to the neck and décolleté area. This is even more important now, since the rise of 'tech neck.' The action of craning our neck to look down at phones and other tech causes creases in the neck and chest to form and deepen, which means that those in their 20s and 30s may require neck products, not just those over 40.

Day
and night

Day ☀

Cleanse in the morning to remove any excess oil, secretion or sweat that built up on the skin overnight. If you want to save time, go over your skin with a TONER on cotton pads, swiped over face, neck, all the way to the hairline and around the ears. If skin is oily, however, a gentle FACIAL WASH is ideal for removing those overnight secretions. If you're the sort of person who likes to jump in the shower first thing, a facial wash or foaming cleanser is a great choice to use then, too, because you can swish it clean away.

You then need to moisturise. Morning products are generally protective, perhaps powered by antioxidants which help to neutralise some of the damage we pick up during the day. After 30 you will probably need a SERUM and/or OIL, but at every age you definitely need MOISTURISER. This moisturiser should sink in well, so that your make-up doesn't slide off. Apply a SUNSCREEN (see p.61).

Now you know what to use, when should you use it? Well, you wouldn't eat the same thing for breakfast as you do for dinner. And your skin, like your whole body, has different needs at different times. The morning is about protection. The evening, replenishment and treatment. But both begin with cleansing.

Night ☾

I talk about your evening cleanse routine on p.55, which I really would like you to do as soon as you get home. Generally, we have a bit more time in the evening, so this is the moment to double-cleanse, then tone, before applying your treatment products.

You'll almost certainly upgrade your moisturiser to a NIGHT CREAM in your 30s. Night treatments tend to be richer and more potent. There are certain high-tech products like retinols (see p.125) that you would only use at night. There are many conflicting studies about the effects of our circadian rhythms on skin, with the debate continuing about whether or not you 'harness' the skin's regenerative powers with overnight treatments, but certainly, anything that's applied at night can get to work at a time when you're in a constant environment, not touching your face or being exposed to UV light.

As a finishing touch, apply eye cream/gel/serum.

Eyes right

I promise that when someone talks to you, they're not noticing your under-eye puffiness, your wrinkles or your dark circles. But because they're high on the list of beauty woes that people mention to me, here are some eye-opening ways to tackle the 'problem'.

EYE BAGS AND PUFFINESS

The reason that eyes get puffed up is that excess fluid collects very easily in this area, which has no bone structure and lots of little sacs that just love to fill up. Several factors make the problem worse: food sensitivities, allergies, your specs resting in the wrong place on your face... as well as too-rich or oily beauty products, which overload the area. After a while, if you don't address the problem, skin may become stretched and crêpe-y, so here's an action plan:

1. **Use a separate eye make-up remover.** Sometimes puffiness can be caused by using your all-in-one cleanser in the eye zone in the wrong way (check your application technique on p.62) or switch to a dedicated product.

2. **Choose the right moisturiser.** Be careful of taking your rich face creams too close to the eye; if you suffer from puffiness, you'll be better off with a lightweight, gel-based eye treatment that sinks in fast.

3. **Massage really helps.** With the right technique, it's possible to get great results massaging the fluid away, physically dispersing the puffiness. A pair of chilled teaspoons (see p.84) or a jade/quartz roller or metal roller designed for the job all help. Use in an outward motion to gently move the fluid out and away, from

just below the eyes, along the cheekbones, towards the hairline. Tapping repeatedly with the right finger along the orbital bone/cheekbone can also be helpful.

4. **For a special occasion, apply a temporary tightening serum.** These can be too drying for everyday use, but may be good as a short-term fix. And if it's a very special occasion you can get quick-fix results from smoothing an ice cube wrapped in gauze over the puffiness in an outwards motion.

5. **Try applying arnica gel to the puffy area.** Massage outward with the technique described above.

6. **Check if your glasses are to blame.** Sometimes ill-fitting sunglasses and spectacles press on the face, causing a 'fluid roadblock'. The same is certainly true if you have to wear protective eyewear in a work setting. Another style or an adjustment may solve the problem.

7. **Drink plenty of water.** It sounds illogical that more fluids would help disperse fluids in the face, but it works. Aim for two litres a day of pure water – not coffee or soft drinks, but water – to help keep the lymph flowing.

8. **When eyes are tired, try 'palming'.** We all spend a lot of time looking at our screens, which can result in eyes that both look and feel exhausted. A technique called palming can deliver soothing results. Place your hands over your eyes with the pads resting on the cheekbone, the fingertips on the forehead. Don't press hard. Close your eyes and spend a few minutes like this; it's a brilliant reset. You can add in a rolling movement from nose to the outside; it's amazing for drainage.

9. **Distract!** Get a great blow-dry. Wear a bright lipstick. Put on some light-catching earrings. You will look fab!

DARK CIRCLES AND SHADOWS

These are often hereditary, and it's fair to say that they can be a tougher challenge than eye bags. Sometimes dark circles are related to your skin tone; if an area has no oil glands, skin can look darker and ashier because of surface dehydration. But never say never; if you figure out the cause of the shadows, you may be able to find solutions:

- **Is it the shape of your eye socket?**
  If you have a hollowed, sunken eye shape, this can create a shadow-like effect. In this case, the fix is a light-reflecting concealer (see p.165). You are aiming to create an optical illusion, as there's no way to change the shape of the eye and your bone structure.

- **Are you just very tired, or have you been ill?**
  Many of us get dark circles when we're exhausted because of, well, life. Overwork, worries, exams, children not sleeping, night shifts... In this case, it's worth investing in a decongesting eye product, such as cooling eye pads, iced compresses or heated compresses that you put in the microwave to warm (these can be super-soothing when you lie down and rest the weighted compress on your eye zone). You want anything that helps with the micro-circulation, which heat and cold do very effectively.

  Tapping massage can help (see p.88). Look for gel formula eye treatments with ingredients such as golden seal, arnica, eyebright and caffeine. Make a point of establishing a good bedtime ritual when you can (see p.320).

Use make-up to distract from the circles: why not embrace the shadow and go with a full-on smoky eye, above and below? Nobody will be able to tell where the smokiness stops and the natural shadow starts. Or go in the other direction, with light and brightness on the top lid. Opt for flesh-toned shades with perhaps a little shimmer, a single tone of shadow or a crayon over the lid that gives full coverage but is paler than your

UNDER-EYE MAKE-UP

Concealer is your best friend here – for men as well as women. We're not talking full, caked coverage, but an imperceptible finish that just brightens the appearance. Before applying, apply a fairly rich eye cream and allow it to sink in for 10 minutes. Apply the concealer but pat rather than stroke it into skin, to layer it on. Use it in a triangle under the whole of the eye, as well as the inner corner of the eye. Also try using some self-tan drops in your moisturiser, or a gradual tanner; this will reduce the contrast between the rest of the face and the shadows so they're less obvious. (Although, I can guarantee they are less obvious to everyone else on the planet than you.) What you're after here, I would say, is an 'improve your skin tone' effect, not 'I'm going to Ibiza'.

dark circle. This is the sort of trick of the light that the Old Master painters used, and it works as well on real faces today!

You can also use tiny touches of highlighter in the inner corner of the eye, on the centre of the top lid and beneath the brow-bone.

Alison's Tip

Consider using retinol products in the form of creams or serums targeted at eyes, to hydrate and gently peel. Hibiscus flower extracts can also be useful, as these contain gentle AHAs (Alpha Hydroxy Acids), to reduce the look of dark circles.

LAUGH LINES AND WRINKLES

Don't use that awful phrase 'crow's feet' to refer to the lines around your eyes. These expression lines – which everyone gets – are there because we've lived, laughed and loved. However, if you'd like to do more than just embrace that, and diminish the appearance of those lines, there's plenty you can try:

- **Rethink where you put your eye cream.**
  Most people tap it onto the eye area of a relaxed face. Instead, smile: you'll see that lines actually extend much further when you do that, in some cases as far as the hairline, and you need to apply your eye product to that entire area.

  If you have crêpiness or sagging (or want to avoid that), you should also apply it to your forehead. Eye sagging begins above the brow, so make sure you treat that area, too.

- **Don't apply eye creams too close to bedtime.**
  Allow a good hour or two for them to start to work their magic, otherwise your pillow will get all those anti-ageing goodies, not your face. If you apply early in the evening, you can double-dose

with a second application and still leave time before bedtime for the product to get to work.

• If one side of your face is more lined, it may be linked with how you sleep.
Most of us tend to favour one side when our head hits the pillow. It's incredibly hard to break that habit, so if you can't manage it, invest in a silk pillowcase or silicone wrinkle patches to reduce the fold. They're a revelation.

• Micro-current treatments can help to firm the eye zone.
You can get eye-specific machines for at-home use (and prices have come right down), as well as salon lifting and firming treatments that target the eye zone. These can be expensive; do ask to see before and after pictures of previous clients, and really quiz the salon on whether those clients had the treatment at that particular salon; sometimes, these can be promo shots issued by the company that makes the machine. If you use a machine at home, you have to be really consistent to get results. You wouldn't expect to go to the gym once or twice a month and see results; it's the same with a facial workout of any kind.

• For a special occasion, try 'face tape'.
There are tapes to lift the eyes, or to apply into the hairline or behind the ears to lift the face and jaw-line. This is the secret weapon of many a Hollywood silver screen goddess, and if you're having a photo taken or you've a big event or birthday coming up, the results can be impressive. But this isn't something you want to experiment with at the last minute – practice makes perfect.

• Use make-up to minimise the appearance of a hooded lid.
There's SO much you can do on the optical illusion front. Whether your eyes are hooded as the result of heredity or the ageing-related crêpiness that some skins are prone to, simply changing where you create your socket line can make a real difference. (See p.202 for

how to create the illusion of an eye socket.) Ditto, having your brows reshaped with a millimetre or two removed under the brow line can lift the appearance of the eye.

If the lids droop, lashes can also start to point downwards, so consider lash perming, lash inserts (applied in salons), or simply switch to a curling mascara that will lift the lashes.

Eye cream how-to

Use a lightweight product if younger, and a richer product if more mature.

1   Dab the product on the two ring fingertips or middle fingertips of each hand (which exert the least pressure on this fragile area).

2   Massage around the brow area (as drooping starts at the brows) and down to the cheekbone in a 'C' movement.

3   Massage the product into the eye socket, following the same 'C' movement.

4   Sweep outwards over the same area to reduce puffiness, from inner socket towards hairline.

5   Smile, to see how far any lines extend; this may be out to the hairline and below the cheekline. Make sure that the whole of the ageing eye area is treated.

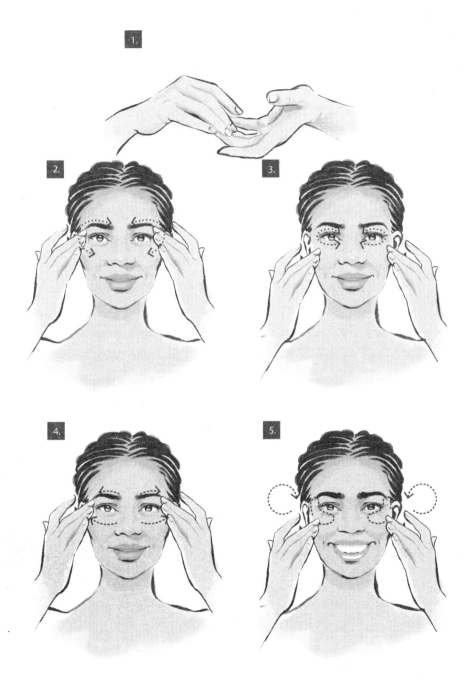

Eye cream how-to: how and where to apply to reduce puffiness and lines

GOING GREEN

In the past few years, the texture and performance of sustainable products has improved beyond all recognition, compared to the early versions of these 'eco' products. There are now organic and natural options for almost every product in your beauty arsenal, and if that fits with your lifestyle and ethos, there are really no compromises that you'll have to make nowadays. Even so-called 'mainstream' beauty companies are making huge efforts to offer refillable products and recyclable packaging, in some cases offering options to return that packaging after use through initiatives like TerraCycle, which upcycles beauty packaging to give it a second life as objects like furniture. At the very, very least, we should all be recycling our own beauty packaging, sorting empties as we do in the kitchen. (There are recycling symbols on the bottom of most packages and jars.)

Why techniques and tools matter as much as products...

Perhaps even more so. Trust me: there's much more you can be doing to get the most out of your skincare choices than just buying products!

- **Up, up, up!**
Always apply cleanser, serum and moisturiser upwards. Your pores are very slightly angled downwards, so in general, all skincare should be applied in an upwards motion, to really get into your pores. In addition, the upwards motion goes against gravity to offer a slight lifting effect, rather than pulling the skin and underlying muscle downwards.

- **Use both hands. Always.**
We all tend to have a dominant hand, but everything you do to your face should use both hands at the same time, to ensure even pressure. That means eye make-up removal, cleansing, toning, exfoliating, moisturising and applying masks. You'll almost certainly need to consciously retrain yourself here. Imagine a line down the centre of your face and mirror the actions with both hands on either side of that line.

- **Break out of the zone.**
If you get a good result from a product, experiment with using it elsewhere. E.g. if you're getting good results from an eye cream, use it on the '11' lines (the frown-lines between the brows), the necklace lines on the neck or the feathery lines around the mouth, and assess improvements. You may well be pleasantly surprised. (Don't do this the other way around; only products formulated for eyes should be used in the eye area.)

- **Way to glow.**

Using a facial self-tanning mist before bedtime or adding a couple of self-tanning drops to your night cream can reduce or even eliminate the need for make-up in the morning, because you'll wake up looking healthy and radiant.

- **Transform any cream into a mask.**

If you have an existing moisturiser that ISN'T quite right for you to use on a daily basis, it doesn't have to go to waste. Consider using it up by slathering it on generously as a face mask, either to be removed with a flannel after a skin-quenching 15 minutes, or leave on as a 'sleeping mask'. Sleeping masks are like face masks that you apply lavishly and allow to sink in overnight, but you can do the same with any (non-SPF) cream. Assess your skin's moisture level in the morning, to check the effect; chances are your skin will be plumped-up and dewy.

Any moisturising face mask can also be left on the skin overnight to hydrate and quench. Avoid doing this with products labelled 'brightening', or clay masks. Just the good old moisturising type.

- **Products only work if you use them.**

Duh! Sounds so obvious. But I've lost count of the number of people who've told me, 'eye creams don't work', or 'neck creams are a waste of money' — yet in reality, they only dip into them once or twice a week, when they can be bothered and/or remember. Look at the manufacturers' instructions as to the frequency (and sometimes the amount) of product to use, and stick to it. You cannot otherwise expect to see any improvements.

- **Don't love a face product? Use it on your body.**

Alternatively, if you have an existing facial moisturiser that isn't quite right for you to use on a daily basis, your body will thank you for lavishing it on arms, legs, feet, ankles and chest. Most people are so bad about decluttering the bathroom cabinet, but this is a good way to use up products and make some space, eliminating guilt at having bought something you are never going to use up on your face.

- **Double-dose neck and chest.**

Take all facial treatments down to your chest and include your chest and neck whenever you moisturise your body. The neck and décolletage is a very vulnerable area, perfectly angled to pick up lots of incidental sun damage, and will really benefit from this product double-whammy.

- **Master the art of the double cleanse.**

If you've been somewhere highly polluted and grubby, if your days are long, if you've been wearing more make-up than usual, or if your skin looks a bit dull, grey or downright 'blah', double-cleansing is a great fix.

One technique is to use two different styles of cleanser. You might start with a micellar water and then follow with a richer oil, cream or balm, which offers slip and glide for your fingers to massage. If you're using just one cleanser, opt for a richer product. I always make the point that your most valuable beauty tools are your hands, but if you lack dexterity or have long nails, you can use a jade/quartz roller, 'Gua Sha' or a facial massage stone. Be lavish and really work the second cleanser into the skin, from your hairline to décolletage. Often, this is all it takes to brighten skin dramatically, in just a few minutes. Remove as usual. It's a good idea to use a warm cloth first and a cool cloth second because it really does leave your skin glowing.

- **Pay into your 'beauty bank'.**

If you know you've got a tough week or a hard day ahead, give yourself some extra TLC. The night before switch off screens, do a double-cleanse, have a long bath if possible, a home facial and/ or some time spent meditating or relaxing, while you can. It's like paying into your wellbeing or beauty bank account so that you can 'draw down' when you're pushed for time.

- **Never let a dab go to waste.**

Any excess face mask, serum or moisturiser should be wiped on the back of your hands, never on a towel.

THE FROZEN SPOON TRICK

Cool, metallic implements are brilliant for massaging the face to depuff, as are jade or quartz rollers. The cooling action takes down the puffiness, but the physical action of draining away fluid is even more important. But metal spoons will also do the trick; I keep spoons in the freezer just for this – smaller for the eyes, larger (tablespoon-sized) for the rest of the face. It feels just so, so good and is just so, so effective for dispelling puffiness.

Frozen spoons for puffy eyes

Apply a little facial serum or moisturiser around the eye area. Using the rounded side of two frozen metal teaspoons, take them from the inner corner of your eye to the temple in an outwards direction, first across the eyelid, then under the eye and over the brow-bone. Smooth them all the way to the hairline each time to massage away puffiness. Repeat for as long as the spoons stay cold.

Frozen spoons for all-over facial massage

I have one of those faces that wakes up puffy; the puffiness goes away as the day wears on, but to fast-forward the depuffing, this is brilliant for making skin icy-smooth and giving a great glow under make-up. It is also good for helping with high colour. You can also do the exact same movements as below with ice cubes, wrapped in gauze to protect the skin.

1   Apply a little facial serum or moisturiser to your face. Using two frozen metal tablespoons, one in each hand, massage your forehead, cheekbones, cheeks, and jawline, in an outwards direction from the centre-line of your face towards the hairline, mirroring your movements on each side.

2   Massage the spoons in a sweeping movement down the side of your face to the bottom of your neck, to help drain fluid away. Repeat as long as the spoons stay cold.

Frozen spoons for puffy eyes

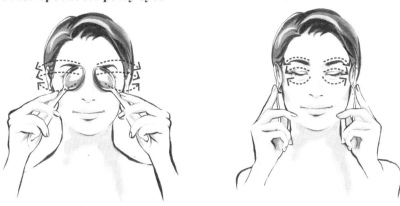

Frozen spoons for all-over facial massage

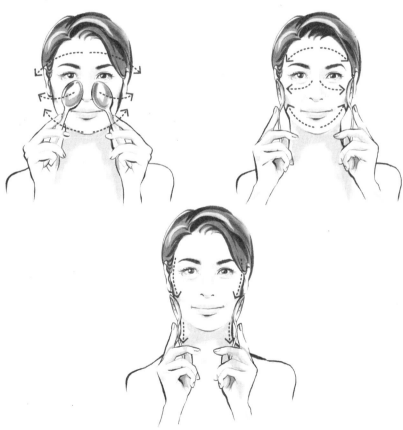

The frozen spoon trick: massaging with frozen spoons to depuff the eyes and face

HAND MASSAGE TECHNIQUES FOR THE FACE

Face massage is the 'secret weapon' of facialists, delivering visible benefits. I like to do them at the second stage of a double-cleanse or before a mask, to get quicker pay-back after a tiring day or week. They really work to 'wake' the face. You can combine these movements with any product that has glide, such as a rich moisturiser, a facial oil or a cleansing balm/oil/cream, to boost radiance, reduce puffiness and/or deliver 'lift'. Once you've mastered these movements, they can be a super-fast way to boost circulation and get a healthy glow back into the skin. Delivered by a professional as part of a facial, they're even better – like an Olympic workout for your face – so if you can, treat yourself every once in a while.

Effleurage

This uses long, sweeping movements of even pressure, via the whole inside of the hands (fingers and palms), ideally with a facial oil or cleanser. Repeat the whole process five or six times and focus particularly on the areas you feel need attention.

1   Mirroring the movements of your hands, massage outwards from either side of the nose and over the forehead, several times.

2   Using one hand at a time, place a hand horizontally on the opposite side of your face and sweep across the chin. Quickly follow with the opposite hand on the other side and repeat several times.

3   Using one hand, then the other, sweep around the face using circular movements – creating a full circle at the outer edge of the face.

4   Using both hands, do some sweeping, lifting movements in an upwards direction on one cheek, then the other.

5   Sweep down the neck, using one hand, then the other several times, to drain the lymph glands.

Effleurage

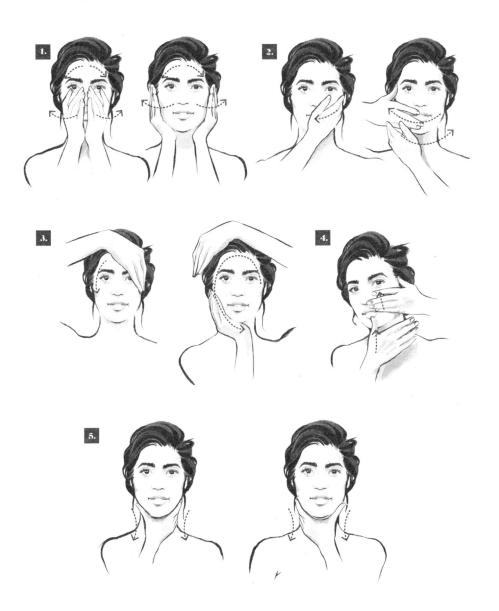

Hand massage techniques for the face

Petrissage

This uses much deeper pressure to reach the muscle layers, boosting blood circulation and delivering a lifting effect, while also destressing the face. Your skin will change colour and become rosier, so avoid if you have naturally high colour. Apply a facial oil or cleanser first and repeat the whole process a few times.

1   Mirroring the movements on each side of your face, use your knuckles to make kneading movements along the jaw line and cheeks, moving outwards.

2   Using your full hands, do some sweeping lifting movements on your cheeks (as for effleurage, but pressing more deeply).

3   Using one hand, then the other, create a cup shape with each hand to apply pressure from the jawline to the lips, giving yourself a 'pout'.

4   Using your fingertips and mirroring your hands on each side of the face, pinch and roll along the brows, lifting upwards. Finish by massaging with small circular movements to drain.

Tapotement

This is a stimulating movement, including (as the name suggests) 'tapping' gestures. You can't use this on skin that is prone to redness, because it brings too much blood to the complexion. But it's great to use before applying make-up or for a tired face at any time; it works on glow and evenness of skin tone.

1   Repeatedly tap all over the face and eye area using your fingertips, as if you were playing the piano, to wake up the skin.

2   Now make 'whipping' movements, almost flicking the skin in an upwards movement – very effective for stimulating blood flow.

3   Tap around the lip area to boost lip fullness; you can also do light 'whipping' movements here, too.

Petrissage

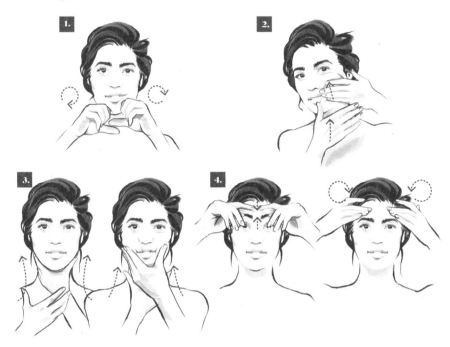

Tapotement

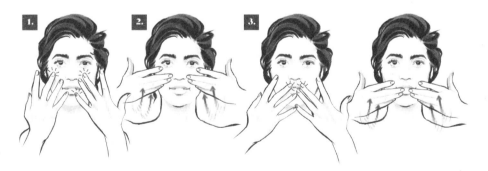

Hand massage techniques for the face

CLEANSING TOOLS

Once upon a time, it was cotton wool or nothing. Now there's a whole 'wardrobe' of cleansing accessories to ensure you get a clean sweep. Here's what to use and why.

- **Cotton wool**

I prefer cotton wool pads to balls, especially the large cotton wool pads which cover a greater area, and are perfect for mask removal. Pads can be used dry (and are highly absorbent), or damp. With some pads you can tease the layers apart; you can then use both layers separately and get twice the quantity out of one packet. Always use real cotton; organic cotton pads are sustainable and widely available. Many old-fashioned cotton balls contain synthetic fibres and skate over the skin; they're useless.

- **Face chamois (or 'shammies')**

These are silky-soft cloths which dry out and actually harden a bit between use, like the chamois you'd use for polishing a car. Because they dry quickly they tend to harbour fewer bacteria. However, I still recommend changing every couple of days and washing on the delicate cycle of your washing machine.

- **Flannels**

Oh, I love a soft, squishy cotton or bamboo flannel. Gentle on skin, but be sure to use a fresh flannel daily to avoid bacterial build-up.

- **Microfibre cloths**

These are made of ultra-fine microfibres which specifically attract dirt and make-up from the face. Manufacturers claim that they work with hot or cold water and there is no need for anything else, but I find that quite a lot of friction is required, especially around the eyes, and I'm not convinced they're such good news for skin. However, they're brilliant if used to remove a cleansing product, and they replace up to 500 single-use make-up wipes.

Alison's Tip

I'm not a big fan of the overuse of cleansing brushes; they over-stimulate the skin if used too often. If you have dry or high-coloured skin they can scratch, and if you have oily skin they can over-stimulate. Cleansing brushes were originally used in clinics for facials, but beauty brands and electrical manufacturers leaped on the marketing opportunity and promoted them for daily use – which is what many users think you should do. Young people with problem skins, in particular, can be tempted to over-use them, in a quest for 'clean' skin, but I believe it's better to dial down and let skin rebalance itself. They are fine for occasional use, as part of a facial, just as you would use a face scrub; they have an exfoliating action (see p.67) so go easy. Sonic brushes are a little gentler than the manual ones.

- **Mittens**
  You can get cloths or flannels sewn into a mitten shape which you might find easier to use.

- **Muslin cloths**
  Now an essential part of so many women's cleansing regimes, but these are not all created equal, and come in varying levels of roughness. Some are so soft that they almost skate over the surface, and don't do a very efficient job. Others can be quite abrasive, sometimes too abrasive, in my opinion, for daily use. If your skin looks red or feels irritated after cleansing, it may not be the cleanser – it may be your cloth. Rough doesn't equal better. Sometimes you have to embark on a bit of trial and error to find the right cloth, among various brands' offerings, but it's important to do that research. Be sure to use a fresh cloth daily to avoid bacterial build-up.

- **Sponges**
  Soft, porous, disc-shaped sponges used to clean skin, gently exfoliating while being super-gentle. They can be synthetic or

BATHROOM MUST-HAVES

Everyone needs these handy, always…

- Hair band/hair ties/clips – for getting all hair off your face

- Dressing gown, so you can change out of your day clothes before your evening ritual. Nothing too precious; you may get product or make-up on it, so it should be easily washable

- Cotton wool pads/washable fabric discs

- Cotton buds

- Spatula or applicator (to stop you dipping your fingers into creams)

- A stack of cleansing cloths or flannels (wash after every use at 30 degrees)

- Hand and bath towels

- Large tissues

natural; konjac sponges are now very popular for cleansing, created from the konjac root, a porous root vegetable from Asia. They can also be used on eyes and are especially good with facial washes. Always wet to soften before use, then wash and dry thoroughly.

- **Tissues**

Good for removing toner or a mask. Go large: buy 3-ply tissues big enough to cover the whole face, and strong enough to press easily onto the face without disintegrating. Be sure the texture's soft and gentle, not scratchy. Never use balm-infused tissues for removing product; they won't absorb anything and you could be allergic to the fragrance.

Skin S.O.S.

Through life, many of us have skin situations that need troubleshooting. We might have temporary flare-ups, our complexions can be affected by a hormonal rollercoaster (teen years, pregnancy, menopause), or as a result of illness. What I've learned – often from first-hand experience – is how to identify and then deal with these challenges.

It can be tempting to throw a lot of money at a 'problem' when that's really not what's needed. On the contrary: that can often make things worse. In general, when you have a complexion problem, you may need to dial down what you do to get back to a state of skin equilibrium. After all, if you've got an upset stomach, would you want rich food? It's the same with skin.

Here is my 'A to Z' of when your skin might need specific troubleshooting help.

ACNE – see SPOTTY SKIN (p.108)

AGEING SKIN

It's inevitable that as we age, the signs of time passing show up. There's generally a natural progression of skin types: oily to combination, combination to normal, normal to dry, and signs of ageing tend to become visible as skin transitions to the dry phase, with lines, wrinkles, slackness and pigmentation. Even if you don't have that many lines, you may clock that your facial contours have changed: your jaw is slacker, for instance, and/or your profile's not the same as it was. This is often a problem with pale skins (because paler skins are more easily damaged by the sun); darker skin tones usually age well.

You may not be bothered in the slightest by signs of ageing – it is, after all, an entirely natural process and it's perfectly OK just to age gracefully, simply ensuring that your skin is well-moisturised, and feeling (in every way) comfortable in your skin. You'll still have lines, but they'll be conditioned, moisturised lines. But you may decide that you want to do whatever you can to make your skin look as good as it possibly can.

To get the best anti-ageing results you'll almost certainly want to be using separate day and night creams (with an SPF for day, for sure), a serum and/or oil plus separate, targeted neck and eye creams. But do also consider electrical implements for facial firming (like electrical muscle stimulation/EMS or red light therapy machines), as these work beneath the skin to stimulate and firm the muscles, as well as boosting collagen and elastin production. On top of your daily basics, a weekly home facial and/or monthly salon facial can pay dividends.

The uncomfortable truth is that ageing skin happens to be the most expensive to look after. You might need to switch to products that contain more potent, perhaps clinically proven, ingredients that address the ageing process: patented molecules, stem cells, peptides, liposomes and retinols. Ageing skin is a sluggish skin, so dial it up: the more you apply, the more ingredients, the more often, with more techniques, more massage and more facials, the better. But you needn't pay the earth; many affordable, high street brands now offer highly effective age-defying creams and treatments.

It's perfectly OK just to age gracefully.

BACKNE

Many people are affected by back acne, sometimes even when their faces are clear of spots. If you've a teenager in the house who sunbathes with a t-shirt on, or who's never seen without a pyjama top, be aware that can be because they're suffering (in silence) from backne. It can last well into adulthood, too.

If the problem's really serious, there are prescription treatments that a doctor can prescribe, to help. But there are plenty of self-help tactics, too. Start by using a skin wash including tea tree, salicylic acid (from white willow) and/or zinc. The challenge with the back area is that it's really hard to reach! If you haven't got someone else to apply it for you, a long-handled sponge can work for application, so long as it's thoroughly rinsed in very hot water and dried between uses, to avoid bacterial infection. Alternatively, a long, thin towel or fibre cloth can be used to apply and lather up the wash. Whatever you use should be soft enough that it doesn't break the skin and spread infection. You can then stand with your back out of the shower leaving the foam and ingredients on the skin to get to work. After showering off, gently pat dry – don't rub – with a soft towel. Again, avoid the kind of friction that can break open a pustular spot.

Follow with a spray toner or a gentle, aromatherapeutic spot treatment that can be misted over your shoulder onto skin, delivering antimicrobial and/or calming ingredients including lavender, tea tree, thyme, lemongrass or oregano. Also try probiotic sprays to help balance the skin.

As an occasional treatment, apply a mud mask with antibacterial ingredients. Arms don't reach the affected area? Apply the mask to a piece of large clingfilm or greaseproof paper (laid on a towel), then lie down on it. Shower the mask off after the prescribed time. Afterwards, apply the sprays named above or a healing gel, such as tea tree or aloe vera, with a ruler if you can't reach.

BLACKHEADS

We all produce sebum – and we need it: it lubricates our skin and is a vital part of the hydrolipidic protective film. Normally, it's invisible: a yellowish clear colour that you don't notice. But when the sebum is blocked in a pore, it thickens, goes white and then it may oxidise and go darker – what we know as a blackhead. Sometimes, people suffer from blackheads as well as spots, but you can just be a 'blackhead person' – they're common to men of all ages; men have more active oil glands because of facial hair growth. Men also often have a simpler skincare regime that may never have addressed the problem of blackheads. (See p.130 for the optimum regime.)

The first treatment tactic is to work your cleanser/exfoliator over the area, focusing gently on the blackheads, with the aim of dislodging the plugs of sebum. Then you could use peel pads instead of toner. That may be all it takes to budge them. (Regular exfoliation helps keep blackheads at bay.) If not, try a targeted mask: many of these are based on charcoal or mud, to draw out the impurities. But sometimes, you need to squeeze – maybe you've got a friend's wedding coming up, or an interview, and just can't live with your blackheads, and there's nothing else for it. Here's the how-to:

- Make sure the skin is clean, warm and softened – perhaps after a bath; it should also be absolutely dry.

- Wrap the ends of your fingers in a tissue so that the skin doesn't get scratched, broken or bruised; the risk, as with squeezing a spot, is that you spread infection. Gently squeeze the blackhead from either side; if it's ready to come out, the oxidised sebum should emerge gently.

- You can buy special blackhead removal tools: long, thin metal implements with a small opening at the end, which can be pressed onto skin and hey, presto! The blackhead squeezes out.

- There are also suction tools, which literally vacuum out the blackhead. They're a bit of a love-hate thing. Personally I've always found it easier to use my hands, but if you're prone to blackheads or have long nails, do try one. If you've got teenagers in the house, it's an idea to leave one of these lying around the bathroom to help them avoid picking at their skin.

Any good facial will incorporate extraction of blackheads; your skin professional can perform these in an expert way, with the help of a magnifying glass (and their years of practice). You might book in as a one-off, or for occasional treatments, if the blackheads boomerang back.

DANDRUFF

Dandruff *is* a skin problem – because your scalp is basically an extension of your face. (Chances are if you have a dry complexion, your scalp will be dry, too.) Sometimes these embarrassing white flakes can just be a short-term problem, so do a little bit of self-reflection, and maybe get your partner or hairdresser to look at your scalp, or take pictures on your phone, zooming in on the area.

Have you been using lots of detoxing shampoos (which can unbalance the hydrolipidic film, if used too often)? Have you sunburned your scalp? Does the list of ingredients in your shampoo feature SLS/SLES (Sodium Lauryl Sulfate/Sodium Laureth Sulfate), which are known to irritate some scalps? Are you using a hair mousse, as these can flake onto shoulders? Are you over-using dry shampoo – as some of these can also flake? Are you over-heating your scalp with a hairdryer? Do you have to wear protective gear on your head, such as a cycle or builder's helmet? Is your comb or brush too sharp, causing microscopic tears on the scalp? Have you been under the weather, which can temporarily cause dandruff?

Lots of questions. But if you've suffered for a while, can't answer 'yes' to any of the above and nothing seems to help, it might be a medical condition, including possibly psoriasis and eczema, in which case consult your pharmacist/doctor or trichologist, if you can access one. If you have redness, soreness, broken skin or any kind of bleeding, then also definitely seek medical advice.

If not, I've a few tricks for you.

- If you have an oily scalp, you can try massaging a mud mask into the scalp, which will help absorb excess oil and clarify the area about 10 minutes before you shampoo and condition as normal.

- If you have dry hair, drizzle a base oil such as sweet almond oil or grapeseed oil directly into the scalp about 15 minutes before bathing or showering and massage it in really well; sometimes, dandruff is caused by the skin cells clumping together, and the massage can dislodge the dried flakes of skin, to be sluiced away as you shampoo and rinse.

- You might also want to check out specific scalp treatment drops, to be drizzled onto hair between washes (without making hair greasy), based on calming ingredients like aloe vera or witch hazel, or declumping ingredients like salicylic acid.

- Switching shampoos can make a difference because they can be formulated with different active ingredients. If you've been using a supermarket brand, or a 'fashion' hair line, look for dandruff treatments from a hairdresser line or a trichologist brand.

- And last, but not least, be sure you're using the correct shampooing technique: a fingertip massage (not the flat pads of your fingers), to stimulate the scalp and lift up hair and massage foam directly onto the scalp, especially the thick area of the crown – with lots and lots of rinsing, afterwards.

ECZEMA

I get so, so many questions about eczema, perhaps because I've never been shy of sharing that I first developed eczema as a child and have learned a great deal about managing it.

Eczema is a form of allergy or sensitivity that can flare up, often apparently for no reason. It can be quite fiendish to go back and try to figure out what was the trigger-point, as it can be caused by so many different things: stress, feeling under the weather, an 'improved' formula

ECZEMA & SENSITIVE SKIN TRIGGER LIST

If you have eczema or sensitive skin, it can be difficult to pinpoint what may be triggering your flare-ups, so here is a list of the (sometimes surprising) things that I have found can set them off. Play detective and really think about whether any of these have changed for you lately, or try taking them out of your routine for a while to see if that makes a difference.

1. Skin products and ingredients, particularly those at the extreme ends of PH scale (remember, the formula may have changed without warning!)
2. Techniques you're using to apply your products
3. New or dirty make-up brushes
4. Unwashed fruit
5. A change in diet
6. A change in your medication
7. Stress or illness
8. Hormonal change
9. Perfume and room sprays
10. Shampoo and hair sprays (as they wash over and fall on skin)
11. Washing powder and fabric conditioner
12. Synthetic and itchy fabrics (such as wool), or new clothes
13. Flannels and cloths you're using on your skin
14. Sun and/or heat
15. Fumes/pollution

of one of your beauty products or washing powder (that's happened to me), staying in a different bed, air conditioning, the fumes in room sprays. (See my 'trigger list' on p.99 for more suggestions.)

There are two types of eczema: dry and wet. The dry type is thickened, reddened, coarsened skin that is cracked-looking. Wet eczema starts to weep and exude. They both tend to itch like crazy – and you need to do everything you can to avoid scratching, which makes things worse. You can get eczema anywhere on the body, but often it can be found in the crevices of the body – elbows, armpits and knees.

As well as seeking medical advice, you can take steps to try to identify what caused it. You should be trying to play detective and figure out any potential causes, while dialling down what you do to your skin and how many products you use. Simplify, simplify, simplify.

Switch to SLS/SLES-free shampoos (see p.236), hand and body washes, as those ingredients are common irritants (they are very drying to skin). The products that you leave on your skin to moisturise and protect it should be very gentle, with short ingredients lists. If your skin is younger and problematic, look for aloe-based products that offer as high a percentage of aloe as possible, because those are closest to this plant in its natural, soothing botanical form. If you have drier skin, choose a single oil to moisturise it – my favourite is rosehip, or try sweet almond, jojoba or olive. Natural ingredients can be very gentle, but be aware that anyone can be allergic to a plant, so don't run away with the idea that plant ingredients are guaranteed trouble-free.

If your skin doesn't improve or flares up, you may need to go down the scientific route, including using prescription products from your doctor.

To conceal, look for vegan-type formulas, including mineral make-up, with its super-short ingredient list.

ILLNESS

If you're sick, concentrating on beating your illness, the last thing you expect or want to have to deal with is changes to skin, hair and nails – yet this is super-common. Skin tends to go haywire first, but hair and nail challenges can show up six weeks or a few months after you've been ill. These changes can last a frustrating amount of time; your skin is the largest organ of the body, and it can take a couple of years for the body to rebalance after serious illness.

Simplify your routine; perhaps return to your go-to 'basic' routine (see p.49). If you notice that you have developed very dry skin, and your normal products sting, dial it down with fewer products, fewer treatments, less often. (The 'single oil' technique for sensitive skin, see p.44, can be good for you, too.) If you've got the energy for a bit of pampering, treat yourself to some beautiful skincare and body care that makes you feel good, perhaps including soothing or uplifting essential oils (so long as those aromatherapy ingredients aren't contraindicated by your treatment – an online search will help you there). Once your skin seems back in balance, post-recovery, you can go back to your regular regime.

Dial it down with fewer products, fewer treatments, less often.

MASKNE

We have all become aware of the realities of mask-wearing and face coverings and they are not good news for skin. A mask creates a 'mini-greenhouse' underneath. When heat builds up, your skin's response is to sweat, upsetting the hydrolipidic film, and one of two scenarios unfolds: skin either goes spotty, or becomes dry, flaky, sensitive and irritated.

If you have to wear a mask for long periods in a work setting, use a cleansing product as soon as you take off your mask, perhaps with a gentle antibacterial facial wash. Keep toner-soaked pads in a plastic bag or container, to sweep over the face and then spritz with a probiotic spray. Remoisturise your skin, again with a probiotic or sensitive skin moisturiser. Use occasional face masks, maybe based around yoghurt, other probiotic ingredients or aloe vera. These are in addition to your normal skincare regime, and can help to get the skin back into balance.

If your skin's become sensitive and you can't use your normal products – perhaps they're causing stinging – then dial down your skincare regime to some really gentle, soothing products targeted at sensitive skin. You might want to use a tea tree toner, or a probiotic mist, but don't use acid-based toners or anything that will strip the skin. Double- or even triple-dose with moisturiser, to get your moisture level up again.

If you're wearing a full visor, you may get blackheads or flaky patches where the mask touches your forehead or rubs against your skin. With elasticated masks, you can get pressure marks where they pull behind the ears. Tone these areas, and replenish with a base oil (such as almond or argan) or a gentle moisturising cream, to keep the area protected and softened.

You may find that you don't want to wear make-up underneath a mask, if you have yours on for long periods. To give yourself a little sweat-proof colour and glow, add a few self-tanning drops to your night-time or morning moisturiser. If you do want to wear make-up, you can look for clay-based products (which absorb sweat and oil) or use one of the newer make-up fixers.

MENOPAUSE

Through peri-menopause and menopause, skin can change quite dramatically, due to hormonal changes. You may develop more pigmentation, dryness, slackening, fine lines and wrinkles, so check out the AGEING SKIN section (see p.94) for detailed info on these. Another challenge is that skin can develop acne rosacea (see p.108).

Hot flushes can trigger shine, so mattifying make-up may be useful at this stage. The sweat produced can cause make-up to slide off your face; try switching to a gradual facial self-tanner or add tanning drops to your moisturiser to give you a hint of a tint that evens out your complexion. Alternatively, one of my favourite tips on the make-up front is to layer up the textures, because this will help them stay put: start with a mattifying primer, then layer on a liquid foundation, followed by cream concealer where needed, then followed by a 'top coat' of powder/mineral foundation for a budge-proof result. You might also like to carry a cooling spritz with you, to take the heat out of skin. Blotting papers or absorbing sponges are best to blot away the sweat. If your scalp is hot and sweaty, try a dry shampoo to prevent or absorb the sweat in the scalp area.

This isn't just about problem-solving; think of this time as an opportunity to reassess your beauty regime and check how it's working for you. If you see a celebrity sailing through menopause in a way that feels impossible to you right now, know that they are probably getting private healthcare and help in numerous other ways. If that sort of help isn't an option for you, remember, what your body is going through is normal, so give yourself a break! Also remember to look after yourself by prioritising sleep (see tips for sleeping through the menopause on p.326), healthy foods and plenty of movement (see the Beauty and Beyond section, p.304).

MILIA

Milia are fatty deposits that have come almost to the skin's surface from within the body to form hard, white lumps. They vary in size from a pinprick to a pea, and they affect all ethnicities. They tend to cluster on the eyes, forehead, upper cheekbones and chin and they can be linked to a health condition, so if you have a lot of them, mention it to your GP. They're not linked with your lifestyle; mostly it's nothing you've done to cause them, although I've seen them quite often on people who don't drink a lot of water. To be honest, though, they're still a bit of a mystery.

You absolutely must NOT attempt to remove them yourself – milia aren't attached to sweat glands or oil glands so there's no 'escape tunnel' for the fat; you will simply bruise, scar and cause infection. One of the gentlest ways to treat them is to massage over the affected areas using your finger, in circular movements, with a tiny bit of oil. This can sometimes help to break up the deposits and disperse them; small electrical massage tools and facial massagers with microcurrents (such as galvanic) can also help. If they are super-close to the surface, peel pads may help, although it may take several weeks of use to see benefits; these are infused with AHAs/fruit acids, and also have a lightly exfoliating texture.

But in general, the most successful results come from an appointment with a professional facialist who will draw out the deposits with a fine needle, or a treatment using lasers or diathermy (high frequency electric currents). If you're nervous about booking, most salons and facialists will offer free, no-commitment consultations where you can discuss your milia to ensure you feel at ease before going ahead.

One last tip, relating to make-up: if you're self-conscious about milia on the top of the cheeks, do steer clear of any glittery and shimmery make-up that will draw attention to them.

PIGMENTATION

Pigmentation is a growing concern for so, so many people. It can take the form of darker, pigmented skin which are also known as liver spots, sun spots, chloasma (especially through pregnancy), or – to give them their medical name – 'solar lentigines'.

These patches of pigmentation can be linked to times of hormonal upheaval, such as pregnancy, as a result of the contraceptive pill, or during peri- and menopause. They can simply be the legacy of time spent sunbathing, perhaps with inadequate sun protection. That damage often shows up years later. Pigmentation can be a side effect of taking antibiotics, which can make your skin more vulnerable in the sun. (Do read medication information; if it says there might be a reaction to the sun, it really means no sunbathing. No arguing. Use SPF 50+ and stick to the shade.)

Yet another cause of pigmentation can be the legacy of acne. Acne scarring doesn't always show as pitting and pock-marking; it may take the form of pigmentation, wherever spots used to be on the face or back.

Areas of pigmentation tend to develop on the cheek area, forehead or the upper lip, as well as the décolletage and (sometimes) on the body, especially hands. If you're concerned, check in with your doctor to make sure they're not related to a medical condition.

Good news: you don't have to alter your whole regime. Address any problem zones with a product formulated with fruit acids, glycolic acid, kojic acid, azelaic acid and/or vitamin C. (The bleaching agent, hydroquinone, has been banned in cosmetics in the EU since 2001 for toxicological reasons and should be avoided at all costs.) These products are often designed to be applied directly to the age spots and pigmented areas themselves, rather than all-over. Anti-pigmentation light therapy machines can also give fantastic results too. But whatever triggered your pigmentation, there is absolutely no point looking at a treatment if you're not going to wear a high SPF (SPF50 or SPF50+), moving forward. We're talking every single day, even in winter; it is daylight – UV exposure – making these marks worse, so you want to shield the skin as much as you can.

A trick of mine is that you can get the best results from using targeted treatments to fade pigmentation during the autumn and winter months, because your skin is *not* being stimulated by the bright light of sunshine. So work on these areas during winter, and by the time spring and summer roll around, those marks shouldn't look so obvious. So long as you remember to keep layering on that SPF…

Switching to natural/ organic make-up brands may help your skin if it's being tricky.

PREGNANCY

The first thing I want to say is: 'Congratulations!' I hope you sail through pregnancy, which for many women is a time when both body and skin bloom and blossom. Not everyone is that lucky, however. And what you need to be prepared for is that it will take two years for your hormones to settle down and rebalance after you've had your baby, so you may experience a rollercoaster situation with your skin, hair and nails between now and then.

You may experience a shift in your skin type. Normal skins may go oily and spotty. Conversely, if you're oily and spotty, you may be delighted to discover that you now have normal, fantastic-looking skin. In some cases, skin may become drier. The key message is not to do anything drastic, because you're at the mercy of your hormones, which is completely natural, and healthy for the baby.

If your skin has no changes, stick with your normal, pre-pregnancy regime. If it's reacting, approach your skin as if it is sensitive (see SENSITIVE SKIN, p.44), giving it plenty of TLC as you count down to the birth and beyond. Just don't overreact; your skin will come back into balance again when your hormones do, but you absolutely don't want to cause another problem by dialling up your skincare regime through adding in more products, more techniques and more ingredients. Switching to natural/organic make-up brands – which tend to have shorter ingredients lists – may help your skin if it's being tricky, too. (See also STRETCH MARKS, p.259, and p.223 for pregnancy hair issues.)

PSORIASIS

Psoriasis appears as silver, dry, grey platelets on the surface of the skin, which is often very red and angry underneath. If you scratch or knock it, it hurts, stings and often bleeds. For some people, psoriasis covers large areas of the body; others have small patches that come and go. Flare-ups can be dramatic and quick.

To be sure it's psoriasis, you first need a medical diagnosis. Take a picture of your flare-ups to show your doctor if you can't get a quick appointment. There are lots of different types of psoriasis, which is a blanket term. I personally suffer from a rare form, psoriatic arthritis, which causes psoriasis flare-ups, both in my body and joints and on my skin. And what I will say from personal experience is that you may not be able to manage the condition – but it *is* possible to manage the flare-ups. Psoriasis doesn't respond that well to cosmetic/beauty treatments, but in addition to following medical advice, there are some tips to follow:

- Read ingredients listings: the shorter and simpler it is, the kinder and gentler your skincare will be.

- Before you get in a bath or shower, lightly massage olive, coconut or almond oil into the affected areas and allow it to sink in. (You can bulk-buy these oils, because you'll be getting through a lot.) Some of the oil will remain on your skin to nourish and comfort it during washing.

- When you wash, use a gentle, SLS-free wash/shampoo to cleanse the body/scalp; any flakes of skin that do come off will be softened and ready to do so.

- I'm not normally a fan of sunbathing, but sensible sunlight can be healthy for managing psoriasis.

- And do, do, do find calming techniques that can reduce your stress levels, as psoriasis definitely flares up when you're stressed, or have other illnesses.

REDNESS/BROKEN VEINS

Couperose, high colour, broken capillaries: whatever name you give to skin that is prone to redness, there's no question it can be very distressing. Sometimes it can be mild; maybe you flush or blush before a job interview or a stressful situation. In this case, a gradual tanner can help even out the appearance of redness, or use tanning drops in your moisturiser every few days, to make it less visible. Do try the calming meditation on p.331, too, because it's often nervousness that leads to this kind of flushing and if you can control your stress levels, that will help.

The next level up is broken capillaries, also known as 'thread veins' or spider naevi, which *aren't* actually broken on the surface but sit just underneath. The watchword here is always 'gentle'. So to exfoliate your skin, avoid physical scrubs, instead switching to an enzyme-based exfoliator or a light peel. Avoid facial steaming, which is a fast track to more broken veins; they're encouraged by extremes of hot and cold, and if you do venture outside in cold weather, add a layer or two of a rich barrier cream to areas where you're prone to broken veins, as extra protection. Spicy foods and excessive alcohol should be off the menu, too, I'm afraid.

Good, concealing make-up can disguise broken veins, and with modern make-up textures, skin can still look very natural, even with a high coverage foundation. The advantage of concealing make-up is that it also acts a bit like an 'overcoat' protecting it from flaring up because of heat, cold or wind.

You might also consider having your broken veins professionally removed by a dermatologist or a salon offering vein removal services, either by sclerotherapy (injecting a saline solution into the skin), or more high-tech treatments (including light treatments). If you're prone to broken capillaries, be aware that these may unfortunately come back elsewhere, a bit like weeds in the garden.

ROSACEA

Acne rosacea goes beyond simple redness. You can get it when you're younger, although it's often associated with menopause, and men can suffer, too. Rosacea may simply take the form of large areas of broken capillaries, but the texture of the affected skin can change, too, becoming lumpy and raised.

If severe or persistent, seek medical advice/treatment. But all of the lifestyle tips for REDNESS/BROKEN VEINS apply. Keep to a simple regime with ingredients that calm and desensitise; don't use too many products and again, look to make-up to give you confidence. You can literally make rosacea disappear to the naked eye with the right make-up; seek out 'free from' products, and do check out mineral make-up (see p.159), which has a very short list of ingredients and can work small miracles.

SENSITIVE SKIN

See p.44.

SPOTTY SKIN

Just because you have spots, it doesn't mean you have acne. It's normal for almost everyone to get a few spots every so often, such as before your period or when you're stressed, no matter what your skin type;

it's to do with the oil glands being a bit blippy, producing more oil at a certain time. Men are also prone to getting them around the beard area. In that case, you can target these with spot or blemish products, perhaps containing tea tree and/or salicylic acid – they should disappear fairly swiftly. Try to avoid harsh, alcohol-based spot treatments.

But if you have skin that is constantly erupting or breaking out, with spots with 'heads' and/or painful, red lumps under the skin, you might need to check in with the doctor, because this is a medical condition. Your acne may be linked with hormonal changes, or the contraceptive pill; hormonal spots are particularly common around the jaw area. Be aware that breakouts can be linked with going on or coming off various prescriptions, in which case, chat with your doctor. Whatever the cause, the doctor may offer you prescription medicines to deal with the problem. I look at teenage skin specifically on p.112.

But there are plenty of things you can do at home. You probably long to clean your skin till it squeaks. But let me tell you: over-cleansing, scrubbing and physically stimulating your skin – perhaps with a cleansing brush – is the very worst thing you can do to it. Dial it all down. Look for a wash-off cleanser with antiseptic ingredients and a gel-based moisturiser. Keep things simple, whatever your age, until your skin rebalances. You want products with short ingredients lists, and as you reduce the number of ingredients and types of products and adopting a gentler rather than a more aggressive approach, you should see a result. For women, the improvement should be visible within a month or so (because of changing oil levels linked to your hormone cycle); for boys and men, sometimes as quickly as a couple of weeks. (If you absolutely have to squeeze a spot, meanwhile, see p.96.)

STRESS

When we're on heightened alert, it affects everything from mental health to our skin, the largest organ of the body. As the stress makes cortisol levels skyrocket, it can impact on the complexion with allergies, sensitivity, rashes or redness. It isn't always that extreme: sometimes, skin goes a little topsy-turvy and you can't quite pinpoint why – but the solution is to dial down your regime and treat skin as if it is sensitive (see p.44), until it rebalances.

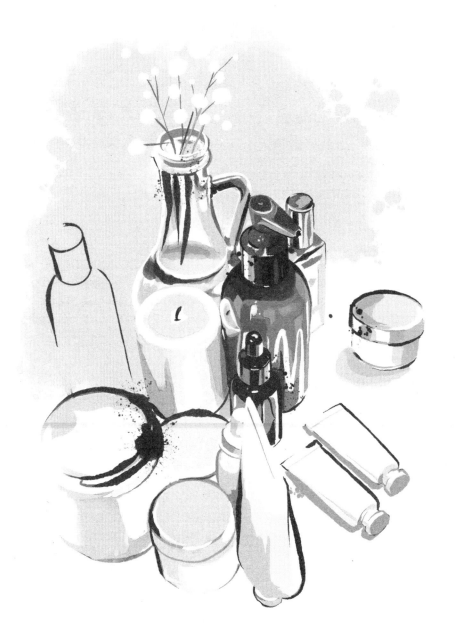

You can't just treat stressed skin from the outside-in though – lifestyle is so, so important. Calm your mind to calm your skin. Here are some tips:

- You need to address your sleep. Stress often causes insomnia, which in turn ramps stress levels up further, so it's a vicious circle. For more on sleep, see p.320.

- Make time to eat regularly and healthily, with lots of fresh foods.

- Cut down on caffeine (or cut it out altogether) if you can – though I admit I'd struggle with this.

- Drink plenty of water. Aim for about two litres a day.

- Practise mindfulness, which I share a technique for on p.331; I bulk-buy a book called *Mindfulness: A Practical Guide to Finding Peace in a Frantic World*, which I give to stressed clients, friends and colleagues because it's the simplest, no-nonsense read and just so, so effective. There is also an audiobook, podcast and app.

- When the world's a whirlwind, you need to centre yourself. You can start to feel very negative about things, and about *you*. What I find helps is to write down positive things to praise about yourself: I got my five fruit and veg – tick! I found a minute to do some deep breathing – tick! I gave myself a facial – tick! I painted my nails – tick!

- And it really is so important to b-r-e-a-t-h-e: sometimes I just do it in a parked car, with my feet on the floor, and breathe deeply and rhythmically for a minute.

I pat myself on the back for all these small achievements, and begin to feel more positive again. Because when the big stuff seems scary, it's important to focus on what we can control, and celebrate these sorts of small wins. I promise: as you calm down, so will your skin.

TEENAGE SKIN

Some sail through the teen years with no major skin problems, in which case a basic cleansing and moisturising routine is all that's needed. However, teen skin is often spotty or acned skin, because of the havoc wrought by hormonal changes from puberty onwards, which result in increased shine (from over-stimulated oil glands), blocked pores and breakouts. Chest, face and back are the common areas. As I've said in the SPOTTY SKIN section, switch to a simple cleansing wash; nothing too heavy, and choose one with antiseptic ingredients like tea tree, chamomile, lavender and aloe vera, which will also soothe and reduce inflammation. Follow with a moisturising gel, not greasy or thick, but something to balance skin and to help prevent scarring – perhaps with propolis, tea tree or aloe in the ingredients list (they're all helpful). Be sure to shield skin with an SPF30+ – look for an oil-free, non-comedogenic formulation that won't block your pores. It's a myth that the sun can improve spots by 'drying them out' – in fact, the opposite can happen because the warmth can stimulate oil production. If you do use a strong, targeted spot treatment, only use it on the spots themselves – not all over! Dab it on with a cotton bud.

If your spots are severe, swollen and you've got more than 15 at a time on your face and back, you may want to visit your GP, who will offer medical solutions. But meanwhile, as a confidence-booster, conceal the spots. That doesn't mean caking on concealer; use a mineral make-up (more about this on p.159), which won't block pores. Or look for plant-based products that will complement your skincare. If you don't want to wear make-up, then a little coat of self-tan is great as it will make the redness less noticeable.

It sounds so obvious, but don't pick – and only squeeze if you must, using the technique on p.96. By being gentle on your skin, you should be able to get through the spotty stage – and it really IS a stage – without scarring.

Calm your mind, calm your skin.

TIRED SKIN

Sometimes, skin just looks as tired as we feel. Dull. Flat. Washed-out. It might appear ashy when you look in the mirror: that's how your skin shows it's lost its vibrancy. It's generally a temporary thing – you've overdone it, need a holiday, have come through a stressful time or are just suffering from lack of sleep or have let things slide with your skincare routine. Skin definitely doesn't look like this when we're back from vacation!

It's time to dial up your skincare regime. What you want is to stimulate your complexion. A quick fix is to double-cleanse for five days. Maybe as a one-off use a facial cleansing brush with a face wash in the shower, in the morning, to rev up your skin. Seek out ingredients with a brightening or glow effect, like enzymes (papaya, for instance), and vitamin C, which is great for radiance. Effervescent, foaming masks are particularly good, and you might use these at the start of the day to wake up your face. You could also add in a course of peel pads to get your glow back. Another fast fix is hyaluronic serum, to quench the skin with moisture. These tactics are good for all skins.

Perk up your skin with make-up (try my glow make-up technique on p.176). Highlighters and colour correctors can work wonders (apricot colour-correctors enliven skin when applied under make-up). Check your foundation shade and finish: could you switch to something with a little more glow/illumination, or a subtly warmer shade? Perhaps you could try a primer with these benefits? You could also mix in a tiny bit of an instant skin tint, while you work towards getting the rest that your body craves.

WHITEHEADS

Whiteheads are tiny white plugs under the skin's surface that happen when oil, dirt and dead skin cells become trapped in pores, generally on the T-zone. In my experience, they're often caused by dirty make-up brushes and tools, or if you don't take your make-up off before hitting the gym or hitting the sack. Or they develop when you apply lots of layers of SPF without cleansing the skin in between; the sun stimulates oil glands and suddenly, you notice you've developed whiteheads.

Whiteheads are generally really easy to clear, so long as you're not harsh with them. Don't pick and poke; instead, use a slightly stronger exfoliant or use a little more pressure when you're exfoliating. Maybe work the area in a circular motion with your scrub and a finger covered in a cloth, and repeat a few days later. Generally, that's all it takes to budge them, but if not try a course of peel pads with mild acids.

Ingredients matter

The beauty world is abuzz with news of both scientific and botanical 'wonder ingredients'. And today, more than ever, we're interested in their power to deliver skin benefits, improvement and tackle challenges. So in this A to Z, I demystify some of the most useful (and talked-about) ingredients, what they can do and who they're best for. This can't be a complete list, so I also encourage you to look at the ingredients lists on your products and start googling! But remember, ingredients are just one part of the skincare story – techniques, frequency of use, gadgets and tools all play a part too – and adding the latest 'trend' ingredient to your regime isn't always the answer. Pay attention to your skin and think about whether you need to 'dial up' or 'dial down' (see p.46–47).

AÇAI

Best for: Mature/dull skin

These deep purple berries are native to South and Central America. The extract is a powerful antioxidant in skincare, featuring brightening vitamin C and vitamin A to boost cell turnover.

AHAs

Best for: Mature/dull/dark skin tones

Found in a wide range of products including cleansers, toners, peels, masks, scrubs and moisturisers, alpha-hydroxy acids (AHAs) work to gently exfoliate dead skin cells from the surface, revealing new, fresh cells beneath, by loosening the bonds that hold skin cells together. These are chemicals, often extracted from natural products, such as glycolic acid (sugar cane), malic acid (apples) and lactic acid (milk).

AMINO ACIDS

Best for: All skins

Amino acids are essential for healthy skin, the building blocks of peptides and proteins. Some are antioxidants and others help the skin to produce its own antioxidant protection, strengthening the skin's immune system and resilience. The amino acids you might see listed include arginine (to restore visible skin damage), histidine (soothing), methionine (protective), lysine (strengthening), and proline and glycine, which work to reduce the appearance of fine lines and wrinkles.

Amino acids are essential for healthy skin.

ANTHOCYANINS

Best for: All skins

You might spot this term in marketing blurb. Derived from plants, these antioxidants – found in cleansers, masks, serums, moisturisers – are blue, red and violet pigments that can protect against UV-induced skin damage. (They are invisible on the skin and won't turn you blue, violet or red!)

ANTIOXIDANTS

Best for: All skins

Ingredients that help guard against the damage done to skin by sun exposure and pollution. Technically, they neutralise 'free radicals'; when the balance of free radicals and antioxidants is out of balance, it results in premature ageing. Antioxidants include vitamins C and E, pycnogenol, resveratrol.

ARGAN OIL

Best for: All skins/dry

Derived from the nut kernel of argan trees, this moisturising oil is sold either as a pure oil or mixed into shampoos, soaps, conditioners, body products, moisturisers, etc. You might think that if you have oily skin, oils aren't for you, but argan oil has an anti-sebum effect and can even be suitable for acned skins.

ARNICA

Best for: Sensitive/reactive skin/inflammation/post-surgery/post-sport

Arnica montana is a herb which is incorporated into creams and gels to reduce inflammation, swelling and bruising. It can also be taken orally, as a homeopathic remedy, for bruising.

ASCORBIC ACID

Best for: Mature/dull/dark skin tones

Also goes by the name l-ascorbic acid, a type of vitamin C that brightens skin, can boost collagen production and protect against free radical damage.

AZELAIC ACID

Best for: Pigmentation/hormonal acne/acne rosacea

This is a natural component of grains such as wheat, rye and barley, and the yeast that normally lives on human skin. A synthetic version is used in cosmetics to help kill the bacteria living within pores, while dialling down inflammation. It can also help to lighten age spots, melasma and other hyperpigmented areas.

BHAs

Best for: Spots/oily/combination/mature/pigmentation

Beta Hydroxy Acids (BHAs), like their AHA relations, can work to smooth fine lines, even out pigmentation and dissolve sticky plugs of sebum and dead skin within pores, making them useful for acne creams, facial washes and peels.

BISABOLOL

Best for: Sensitive/acne/rosacea/redness/mature skin

A soothing chamomile extract with antimicrobial and anti-inflammatory actions. It also helps other ingredients (such as oils, vitamins and minerals) to penetrate deeper into the skin, and has been found to stimulate collagen production.

CANNABIDIOL (CBD)

Best for: Mature/dry/acne/eczema/hormonal acne/acne rosacea

A 'buzz' ingredient derived from the hemp plant, a member of the cannabis family, with the psychoactive elements stripped out, CBD oil is safe to use topically. It is anti-inflammatory, antioxidant and anti-ageing. Look for products that mention 'cannabidiol', 'hemp extract', 'broad-spectrum CBD', 'full-spectrum CBD' or 'hemp CBD' on the label; hemp seed oil is from a different part of the cannabis plant and does not have the same actions.

CERAMIDES
Best for: All skins

Naturally occurring lipids found within the skin's serum and mimicked in skincare, to help moisturise, nourish and restore the skin's barrier.

CICA
Best for: Mature/sensitive

Centella asiatica is derived from tiger grass, and has been used in Chinese medicine and skincare for decades, but products featuring this moisturising ingredient have been 'rebranded' as CICA creams, to create a buzz around them. Antioxidant and anti-inflammatory, it helps repair the skin's barrier and firms, smooths and targets lines and wrinkles.

COCONUT OIL
Best for: All skins/dry/sensitive

Could be taken as (literally) a desert island product, this saturated fat – which is easily found on supermarket and natural food store shelves – can work as a cleanser, moisturiser and hair treatment. It is liquid when warm, solid when cold (a cool bathroom is enough to solidify it) but it melts at body temperature and is a versatile, nourishing, multitasking top-to-toe treat.

COENZYME Q10
Best for: All skins/ageing

A powerful antioxidant (also known as ubiquinone), particularly widely used in products targeting fine lines.

COLLAGEN
Best for: All skins/dehydrated/ageing

Within the body, collagen helps build strong skin, bones and muscles, but production slows down as we age. The molecules are too large to penetrate the skin when applied to the surface, so you can't top up your collagen levels by applying it externally, unfortunately; the best thing you can do to preserve your skin's own collagen level is to apply sunscreen.

However, topically applied plant collagen is great for plumping up the appearance of your skin.

Electrical stimulation treatments can boost collagen production, but you'd need a series of these (and they're expensive) to see a difference. You could invest in a home-use machine, but you'll have to use this daily for a few months.

COPPER PEPTIDES

Best for: Mature/sensitive

These are amino acids with an antioxidant action, found to promote collagen and elastin production within skin, but are most efficient as a catalyst to help other ingredients to absorb.

DIHYDROXYACETONE (DHA)

Best for: All skins, for self-tanning

The most widely used active ingredient in topical tanning products, often derived from sugar cane or sugar beet. This colour additive reacts with the dead cells on your skin's surface to darken it, faking a tanning effect that fades after a few days.

DIMETHICONE

Best for: Oily/combination skin/haircare

One of a family of silicones, which are slippery ingredients that hydrate and protect the skin, with a smoothing effect. Dimethicone often features in oil-free moisturisers and skin-smoothing primers, and is also widely used in haircare.

ENZYMES

Best for: All skins

Enzymes from ingredients like papaya, pumpkin and pineapple have a mild exfoliating action, breaking down keratin proteins in the cells (although this sloughing is invisible to the naked eye). Enzymes are generally tolerated by fragile skins that find scrubs too sensitising.

ERYTHRULOSE

Best for: All skins for self-tanning

A sugar-derived self-tanning agent extracted from red berries, often used in combination with DHA (dihydroxyacetone) to create a fake tan that fades within a few days as the surface cells slough away.

ESSENTIAL OILS

Best for: All skins/multiple uses

Essential oils are valuable, minute drops of concentrated oil extracted from plants. The most concentrated solutions are known as 'absolutes'. Some of the benefits of essential oils can also be found in the liquids produced as a by-product of their extraction, such as rose water. Essential oils are some of the most powerful ingredients and they're also complex; each oil can have over 100 chemical components. Each plant extract has different effects as a topical application and when inhaled. For example, rose is anti-ageing when applied to the skin and calming when inhaled; ylang ylang is good for oily skin and considered an aphrodisiac; lavender is used on sensitive skin and to encourage sleep. As a trained aromatherapist, I could write a whole book on this!

GLYCOLIC ACID

Best for: Mature/pigmentation/acne/skin resistant to other treatments

Available in washes, lotions, serums, peel pads, spot treatments and face washes, glycolic acid is an AHA derived from sugar cane – one of the more powerful fruit acids available. It's particularly useful at both ends of the age spectrum: on acned skins it can improve the appearance of both acne and acne scarring, through a peeling action. (Research has shown it also has an antioxidant and antibacterial action.) On mature skins, it can have a brightening action, diminishing sun spots, reducing fine lines and increasing the thickness of skin, as well as helping to even out skin tone. But it's not without risks: be aware that if you have dry or sensitive skin or a dark skin tone, some glycolic products can cause problems, and whatever your skin type, proceed with caution while you establish how your skin reacts; it won't suit all. A high SPF is essential when using glycolic.

Hyaluronic is every skin type's best friend. You literally can't overdo it.

HUMECTANTS

Best for: All skins

Hyaluronic acid (see below) and glycerine are examples of humectants, useful because they actually pull the moisture from the air around us, and into the top layers of skin from beneath, holding moisture from topically applied products to improve hydration.

HYALURONIC ACID

Best for: All skins

You'd have to have been living on Mars not to be aware of this ingredient, as there's been a huge buzz about it in recent years (I've been a fan for 35 years!). Hyaluronic acid is present in the cells of our own bodies, vital for keeping moving parts and fluids viscous. As a molecule, it can be applied to skin, working as a humectant. It has an extraordinary power to hold about 1,000 times its own weight in water, keeping skin hydrated and plumped up. What often puts people off is the term 'acid': it's easily confused with exfoliating acids like lactic, glycolic and salicylic, all of which need to be added to a routine more sparingly and carefully. But hyaluronic is every skin type's best friend, to be found (and enjoyed) in creams, serums, lotions, tonics, mists, body products and foundations. You literally can't overdo it and it can work wonders on dehydrated and ageing skin. I cannot recommend it enough.

KAOLIN

Best for: Oily/combination

A clay, found in masks, make-up and some washes, which absorbs oil and reduces shine. It can be used by other skin types but may feel drying.

KIGELIA

Best for: All skins

Also known as the 'sausage tree' (from the shape of the fruits), cultivated in Africa, *Kigelia africana* has antimicrobial, skin-toning properties and may prove helpful for eczema and psoriasis.

LIPIDS

Best for: All skins

These are naturally present in the body, present in the upper layers as sebum, as well as natural ceramides, cholesterol and fatty acids. Think of them as the body's natural lubrication. Some skincare ingredients (including CERAMIDES) are referred to as lipids; they lubricate from the outside in.

LIPOSOMES

Best for: All skins

Liposomes are encapsulated ingredients (tiny sacs) which are 'launched' into the skin – a little like tiny rockets containing their skin-caring cargo. They allow ingredients to be delivered a little more deeply.

LYCOPENE

Best for: All skins

This antioxidant red pigment is found in watermelon, tomatoes and carrots, and can help to protect skin whether you apply it externally – most usually in a moisturiser or serum – or eat it (either in the form of those fruit/vegetables, or as a supplement).

MANDELIC ACID

Best for: Acne/oily/sensitive/mature/pigmentation

Derived from bitter almonds, mandelic acid is gentler on skin compared to other AHAs (alpha-hydroxy acids), making it less irritating to sensitive skins. Useful for dark spots, dullness, wrinkles, acne and acne scarring.

MANKETTI OIL

Best for: Dry/oily skin/textured hair

Also known as mongongo oil, from the nuts of mongongo trees (which can withstand drought and wide temperature swings). A very emollient oil, rich in Essential Fatty Acids (EFAs), it helps unblock pores on the scalp, while also nourishing textured hair.

MARULA OIL

Best for: All skins

Extracted from the fruit of marula trees, this is a swiftly absorbed oil high in EFAs and antioxidants.

NANOSPHERES

Best for: All skins

Another word for tiny, spherical particles, which can penetrate more deeply into the top layers of the skin than many ingredients.

NIACINAMIDE

Best for: Mature/pigmentation

A type of vitamin B3 (niacin) which strengthens the skin's outer layers, boosts elasticity and soothes redness and irritation; it can be helpful for acne, rosacea, hyper-pigmentation, fine lines and wrinkles.

OXYGEN

Best for: All skins

Oxygenating skincare has its origins in medical treatments; pressurised oxygen is used in hospitals to kickstart or speed up the healing process of burns. Oxygenating skincare – generally masks, which bubble or foam painlessly on the skin – can help to boost cell metabolism so that dead cells are shed and fresher cells become visible, leaving skin brighter-looking.

PARABENS

A controversial family of preservatives which can, in some cases, be irritating to sensitive skins or those with eczema or psoriasis. The jury is still out, for me. On the one hand, there have been countless 'scare stories' about these ingredients (they have weak, oestrogen-like properties), but on the other, many studies claim that they're completely safe; they have been approved by authorities for safe use in cosmetics, and are found in many convenience foods.

However, knowing that many beauty shoppers try to avoid them (whether or not their fears will ever turn out to be founded in science), many brands have moved away from using them in recent years. If parabens do feature in a skincare product you use, do know that they are there in absolutely minuscule quantities, right down the ingredients list.

PARFUM

This is fragrance, usually a complex mix of hundreds of different scent components, and you don't want to see it high up an ingredients list, as it's a potential skin irritant. Near the end of the list means it's there in a small quantity, so less likely to cause a problem. Try to avoid it completely if you have sensitive skin.

PLANT STEM CELLS

Best for: All skins/anti-ageing

In nature, plant stem cells are clever things: they have the ability to divide and boost growth in any part of the parent plant. Plant stem cells, for instance, from apple trees or melon plants, have been turning up more and more in beauty products in recent years, as an anti-ageing ingredient, targeting lines, cross-hatching and crêpiness.

POLY-HYDROXY ACIDS

Best for: All skins/sensitive

PHAs, for short, are considered 'cousins' of AHAs and BHAs, with a similar skin-brightening action as they chemically exfoliate the skin. The most common are gluconolactone, galactose and lactobionic acid. They work only on the surface as they can't penetrate as deeply as AHAs and BHAs, and may be less irritating, so more suitable for sensitive skins.

PREBIOTICS/PROBIOTICS

Best for: Acne/sensitive skin

We're starting to understand much more about what probiotic creams can do for the skin. *Prebiotics* are a bit like fertiliser or food that can help certain good bacteria to flourish. *Probiotics* are beneficial strains of live bacteria, either taken orally via supplements or fermented foods (kimchi, sauerkraut, kombucha etc.), or applied to the skin via mists, creams and serums to improve skin health. Certain strains can be particularly good for acne, others for sensitive/reactive skin. They are especially good if skin is out of balance from excess sweating, e.g. sport, wearing masks or hormonal flushing.

RETINOIDS

Best for: Acne/mature

The general term for all vitamin A derivatives to be found in skincare. It's a 'trend ingredient' that's come back and many brands are trumpeting that their natural ingredients – such as carrot and rosehip oils – contain retinoids, but be aware that these are not as potent as scientific concentrates. See Retinol, below.

RETINOL

Best for: Acne/mature

Retinoids such as retinol (in over-the-counter products) or tretinoin and Retin-A (prescription only) help skin to speed up cell production, working to push out/slough off dead cells, unclogging pores – which is why they're useful for spotty skins and large, open pores.

On mature skins, retinols work effectively to smooth skin, tackling pigmentation, fine lines and wrinkles.

At whatever stage of life, be aware these are potent ingredients and need to be introduced gradually, starting with low levels and used at intervals; retinols can result in irritation, dryness, redness and flaky skin. Because retinols slightly thin the skin, they make it more vulnerable to sun damage; always apply a high factor SPF30 or SPF50, even if it's cloudy outside.

My first choice on an overactive, spotty skin is a calming regime, see p.108. However if you get limited results with this, step up to retinol, but proceed with caution due to the reasons above.

SALICYLIC ACID

Best for: Oily/spots

A type of BHA, or Beta Hydroxy Acid, from willow bark. It is oil-soluble, which means it can penetrate into oily pores, and is used as a chemical exfoliant in products targeted at acne.

SULPHUR

Best for: Oily/spots

Sulphur works to dry out the surface of skin, absorbing excess oil that can lead to breakouts. It's naturally antibacterial and anti-inflammatory, helping to prevent new bacteria from colonising the skin's surface. Not so good for dry and sensitive skins.

THALASSOTHERAPY

Best for: All skin/dehydrated/sensitive/ageing

This term is sometimes used for spa treatments that use sea water, but also incorporates a large group of skincare ingredients based on thousands of different seaweeds and sea mineral extracts. They're used mainly for their hydrating and balancing effects, but when combined into more sophisticated formulas they can also have great anti-ageing benefits too.

TITANIUM DIOXIDE

Best for: All skins

A pulverised mineral which works as an effective sunscreen. It's what's known as a 'physical sunscreen' ingredient, because it sits on the surface, bouncing UV light off skin, and is tolerated by skins that may be irritated by chemical sunscreens. It's ground into teensy particles which are mostly invisible to the naked eye, although some physical sunscreens do make skin look a little ghostly.

VITAMIN A

See RETINOIDS/RETINOL.

VITAMIN C

Best for: All skins

A powerful antioxidant that helps prevent and treat UV-related ageing, including pigmentation. It's a very unstable molecule that breaks down quickly if exposed to air and light, but formulators have got much better in recent years at ensuring that vitamin C stays active in a formulation (look for the words 'anhydrous', 'encapsulated' or buy in its powder form, to ensure that it is active). It appears on labels by many different names including L-ascorbic acid (often referred to as ascorbic acid), magnesium ascorbyl palmitate, etc. but generally, brands will shout out the fact a product contains vitamin C.

VITAMIN E

Best for: All skins

Also known as tocopherol, this is another powerful antioxidant vitamin which can help guard against UV damage to skin, protecting it against free radical damage. It is used both as a cosmetic ingredient, in almost any kind of formula (even make-up), and a nutritional supplement, to work from the inside out.

WATER

Best for: All skins

Very often top of the ingredient list in a product, used – in distilled, purified or deionised form – as the basis of many liquids, creams and gels.

ZINC OXIDE

Best for: All skins/acne/rosacea

From zinc, a mineral found in nature. Tiny (nano) particles of zinc are formulated into physical sunscreens to shield skin by bouncing light from the skin. It' also used in products for treating acne, rosacea and dandruff.

pH

The skin's surface is naturally slightly acidic, with a normal pH of 4.7 to 5.75. Oily skin is at the more acidic end of that range and dry skin is at the more alkaline end. Men's skin tends to be slightly more acidic than women's.

Skin has a protective film called the acid mantle or hydrolipidic film, which works with other elements present (cholesterol, enzymes, sweat, ceramides and oil) to protect the skin. The pH works to keep this microbiome balanced. If you disturb the skin's pH too often, it can lead to various problems. For example, most soaps are alkaline, which is why you tend to get a tight, dry feeling from washing with bar or liquid soap. The vast majority of skincare products are 'pH neutral', which means they are formulated with a pH balance of 4 to 7, compatible with the skin. However, as you can see from the diagram opposite some of the stronger 'trend' ingredients we're using today sit outside our normal range. Bear in mind, these products promise certain actions but but they also carry a stronger risk of reaction. They can have the effect on skin we're looking for (such as anti-ageing) but for some they can also cause sensitivity or other problems, as they are not always suitable. So go carefully, and 'dial it down' if this happens to you (see pp.46–47).

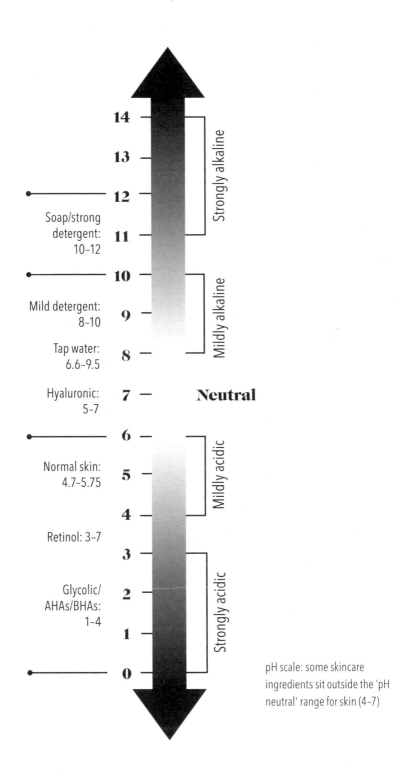

14 — Strongly alkaline

13

Soap/strong detergent: 10–12

12

11

10 — Mildly alkaline

Mild detergent: 8–10

9

Tap water: 6.6–9.5

8

Hyaluronic: 5–7

7 — **Neutral**

6 — Mildly acidic

Normal skin: 4.7–5.75

5

4

Retinol: 3–7

3 — Strongly acidic

Glycolic/ AHAs/BHAs: 1–4

2

1

0

pH scale: some skincare ingredients sit outside the 'pH neutral' range for skin (4–7)

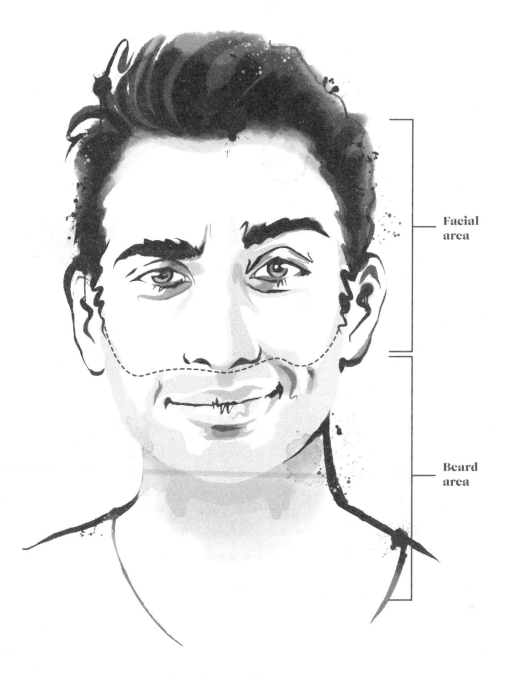

Facial
area

Beard
area

Men's skin can be divided into two areas

For men only

Male skin needs a two-way approach, and probably, more TLC than it's currently getting...

For the vast majority of men, daily routine skincare – over and above tackling a beard – is a fairly recent discovery. Growing up, the priorities tend to be dealing with spots and establishing a shaving routine. Anti-ageing or even 'comfort in a jar' may not have been on the radar, yet skincare is just as crucial for men as women. Increasingly, men are becoming interested in having a grooming/beauty routine, so you will find many sections of this book relevant – all the previous information on skincare is relavant to you too.

However, men's skin does have some differences to women's skin. Men tend to age differently from women – and often better. Think of the male face divided into two halves: the beard area (from cheekbones, all the way down the neck), is well served by oil glands and benefits from their natural, age-protective action. The skin above is more like a woman's, with fine lines and wrinkles appearing around eyes and forehead, and perhaps dark circles beneath the eyes. Here's how to give male skin the care it needs to look its best, for both areas of the face.

- **You CAN get away with just shaving.**
  How you do that is entirely up to your preferences. It's about performance: finding the product that gives you the closest shave. If you haven't tried one, you might want to try a **shaving oil.** Massaged into skin before shaving, a shaving oil plumps up the skin and improves razor glide, while moisturising the area to help prevent razor burn and rashes. You can also use facial oils for this. If you like to use a foam shaving product, try a light layer of facial oil underneath to 'buffer' skin from the drying effect of the foam and the scraping of the blade, helping to prevent shaving rash and soreness.

If wet-shaving, always shave downwards. That will help prevent ingrown hairs, razor lumps and bumps. If you do get problems with rashes and lumpiness in the beard area, try switching from 'fashion-led' products (fragrance-led, or perhaps endorsed by a celebrity) to products from skincare brands which are specifically designed to calm, desensitise and prevent problems.

Be aware that traditional splash-on aftershaves are based on alcohol; if you've been conditioned to think that that stinging sensation is manly, it's not! It's damaging and drying to skin. Apply aftershaves, colognes and fragrances to chest, arms and back of neck only, although never before sunbathing as they can sensitise the skin and cause pigmentation marks.

• Cleanse skin daily.

A **facial wash** can be used in the shower or before/after shaving, to remove excess oil and bacteria. This is especially important if you have a beard or stubble, where high germ levels have been observed! You may also enjoy the occasional deeper cleaning action of a **cleansing brush**. If you're clean-shaven you can experiment with other types of **cleanser** such as balm, cream, lotion, etc. (see pp.48–53).

Add in an occasional exfoliating **scrub**, to buff skin and prepare it for serum and moisturiser (see p.67–69). What's the main difference between male- and female-focused skincare ranges? Packaging. Choose whichever works for you.

You could also try using **toner** – a spritz-on mist or a toner applied from a bottle on a cotton pad; this removes the last traces of wash/cleanser and helps 'prep' the skin for the next step.

• If you're looking fatigued, eye products can help.

There are many anti-fatigue **eye treatments** (gels and creams) available which target dark circles and eye puffiness, often with subtle illuminating ingredients that work to brighten the area without being visible. You only need a tiny amount, literally, a dot the size of a grain of rice, per eye. (If you overload the eye area, you'll get puffiness.) A **concealer**, meanwhile, can cosmetically disguise dark circles and freshen the face.

- **Above the beard area, a man's skin is similar to a woman's.**
So if you want to prevent or treat fine lines and wrinkles, add in a **serum** product with anti-ageing benefits, and use it from the beard-level upwards. If your skin is very dry, an additional **moisturiser** (applied after a serum) can be really soothing and comforting, as can a facial oil used all over, or an aftershave balm.

- **Try a mask or facial.**
Many salons, hotels and spas now offer specific menus of men's treatments (and there are even men-only salons), to tackle challenges such as blackheads around the nose. A facialist will perform 'extractions', to remove these. These facials can be a great way to discover new products and whether you like the fragrance or feel of them on your skin, as well as receiving a personal expert recommendation for the products ideal for you. (On the other hand, don't feel you HAVE to buy anything.) **Face masks** for use at home can boost hydration and give a natural-looking glow, or decongest skin, perhaps via clay or charcoal ingredients.

- **Don't dismiss the idea of make-up.**
I applaud a guy in full make-up, but if that's not you it can still offer subtle ways of looking healthier. **A tinted moisturiser** can effectively even out skin tone and add a healthy glow. Or try 'invisible' make-up, via a gradual face tanner or by mixing self-tanner half-and-half with a moisturiser, then smoothing into the whole face and neck. Tanning drops have the same effect, and the results are imperceptible. This 'can't-tell-it-from-real' glow doesn't wash off but gradually fades, over a few days. Top up as you like.

Ask Alison: skincare Q&A

Here are the answers to skincare questions I get asked time and time again…

Q: How do I use sunscreen within my facial regime?

If it's sunny weather or you're on holiday, sunscreen is your No.1 morning priority. Apply a once-a-day sunscreen or a repeat application product, at least 30 minutes before going outdoors. Any complex skincare (serums, creams etc.) should be moved to the evening, so you can focus on the all-important safety factor of SPF. If you're repeat-applying during the day, sweep a toner-soaked cotton pad over your face first. You should also stay in the shade as much as possible! (Ideally, your sunscreen replaces morning moisturiser, so find a texture that's rich enough for you. If you can't find an adequately moisturising formula, use your normal moisturiser first, but allow 10 minutes for it to sink in before layering on the sunscreen.)

If the weather is dry and windy, one of my tricks is to use a once-a-day SPF first thing, but a repeat application SPF throughout the day, to top up the skin's moisture level.

Sunscreen is removed at night just like any other facial skincare, through your normal cleansing routine.

Q: How can I tell my skin type?

Your skin type is determined by the level of oil production. You can gauge your skin's natural oil levels by peeling a facial tissue down to one layer and pressing it firmly onto make-up-free skin. Leave it there for a few minutes and remove; if you have oil on the tissue pretty much all over where it touched your skin, your skin is oily. If you have oily patches on nose, chin and forehead, you're combination. Anything else is dry or normal. A good time to do this is a couple of hours after your morning or evening skincare routine when products will have been absorbed, so not overly present on the skin's surface.

Q: What is the difference between a skin type and a skin condition?

A **skin type** is fixed for years at a time. It can change during times of hormonal change, and due to ageing (see p.35).

A **skin condition** can arise really quickly, almost overnight, sometimes as a reaction to a product, for instance sensitivity to a too-strong ingredient. Using products to tackle a skin condition takes precedence over your normal skincare routine (see p.44).

Sometimes you might *think* your skin has changed and become oilier overnight, but it's more likely due to hot weather or exercise. Oily skin is oily morning, noon and night.

Q: I have a dark-toned skin – what SPF do I need?

It's an absolute myth that dark skin tones don't need sunscreen; you should still wear an SPF30 or above, on your face. Check the formulation because some sunscreens based on titanium dioxide or zinc look ghostly on all skin tones, but may be more visible on yours. Redness is a sign of obvious damage on skins, but skin is also exposed to UVA rays, which are the ageing rays. (Think of them as: UV-Ageing, UV-Burning.) Sunscreen also guards against the increased likelihood of long-term skin changes which may result in skin cancer.

Q: My skin has suddenly aged quickly – what can I do?

We all have ageing spurts, as we had growth spurts when young. Sign yourself up to skincare 'boot camp' and 'dial up' your routine, adding in some anti-ageing products (serums, lifting creams, lifting eye products). Start layering your products (see p.139). What also works wonders is to firm up the 'facial architecture' – the underlying muscles – using electrical machines that give them a workout, using electrical microcurrents/faradic currents, literally like a 'face gym'. Light therapy and laser therapy can also be helpful. All of these technologies have trickled down to at-home use devices, so these are no longer salon-only options.

Q: I've recently lost weight and my face looks gaunt. What to do?

Your skin is the body's 'envelope' and when it's full, the fat cells are plumped up and the skin looks smooth. When you lose weight, you don't lose fat cells but they shrink and the envelope droops, resulting in slackening. Switch to anti-slackness/firming products in terms of your moisturisers and serums, and turn to electrical devices (see above) to firm the underlying area; this stimulation can also work to boost collagen and elastin production. You could also look at new make-up techniques that can help 'lift' (see MAKE-UP CHAPTER). Also, why not speak to your hairdresser for a new cut or style to flatter your face shape.

Q: I've lost weight but my face is feeling very dry. Any ideas?

If you've been on a low-fat diet, this often manifests as dryness because the body needs healthy fats, and when it doesn't get them, it shows up on the largest organ of the body, your skin. Even a previously healthy skin can appear very dry on a low-fat diet. Taking a balanced essential fatty acids supplement can be helpful, so have a go and see if that improves things. You can also up your programme of exfoliation, and get butters and oils into your skin; this is the time to embark on weekly facials, and smooth in overnight rich masks. Try my Instant glow make-up on p.176–77 using creamy and buttery textures in your make-up, too.

Q: My skin is so dry that nothing seems enough. What can I do?

Dry skin holds onto dead skin cells. You need to enrol it into 'skincare boot camp', exfoliating those dead cells by scrubbing gently several times a week, then layering up moisturisers to top up moisture levels. Keep moisturiser handy: put a jar on your desk or keep it in your work locker, to apply during the day if you're not wearing make-up. Keep a pot by the bed or loo so that when you get up in the night, you can reapply moisturiser in the dark! If the dry skin is all over your body, shower with oil massaged in beforehand.

Q: I always look tired – what can I do?

Switch to products which promise 'glow' – honestly, the clue is often in the product name! Look for words like 'luminising', 'glow' and 'radiance' and move away from matte or velvet-finish make-up. Choose 'luminous' primers and foundations, or add glow drops to your regular foundation, which make skin appear revitalised via light-reflecting pigments (and often pack a skincare punch, too). To awaken the look of the skin itself, also quench it with masks and try adding a vitamin C- and hyaluronic-based product to your skincare, which work to brighten and plump.

Q: I've been dieting but my skin's gone very spotty...

I often find that when people start dieting, they start juicing or eating a lot of extra fruit, which is introducing acid into the diet, resulting in spotty skin. A spotty skin is more acid naturally, so by increasing acid in the diet, it tips the balance. Increase 'neutral' vegetables in your diet such as carrots, cauliflower, lettuce, red cabbage, avocado, beetroot, broccoli, leeks and cucumbers – and opt for green/veg-based smoothies rather than fruit-based. You can also dilute them with some water.

Q: I'm going on holiday. What are the essentials to take? I don't want to take everything!

If you just want to pare back to the minimum, this should still cover it!

- **Cleansing bar** (which will do face and body and doesn't count as an in-flight liquid)

- Bottle of **tea tree** oil which multitasks as an antiseptic

- **Deodorant**

- **Insect repellent (with DEET)** and **bug sting treatment**, for hot countries

- **Once-a-day sunscreen**

- **Moisturiser** that is dual purpose for face and body. If you choose an aloe vera-based product, it can serve as aftersun too

- **Shampoo** that doubles as a shower gel

- **Conditioner.** Then you're good to go…

Personally, though, I go in the opposite direction for holidays! I like to make the most of the fact that someone else is cleaning the bathroom and washing the fluffy towels, so I pack lots of different beauty products and make time for face masks, to work on hands and cuticles, use different moisturisers and body creams/oils… If there's no counter space in the bathroom, I lay them all out on the table in the bedroom and I love taking time for pampering while I'm away.

And one of my tips is that if you want to take a lot of products, pack them in a golf bag or sports bag, even if you don't play that sport. You might like to know that these over-sized bags are charged by the bag not by the weight so you can pack it with extra (well-wrapped) cosmetics. (Until they read this in which case my trick is foiled!)

Q: What are the side effects of retinol? I think I might have a reaction…

Retinol (see p.125) is easily available now, widely used as an anti-ageing ingredient (see p.94). The commonest reaction to 'beauty retinol' (as opposed to doctor-prescribed retinol) is that skin can go a bit flaky and red, or become spottier. Always introduce retinol gradually – one night on, two or three nights off, then every other night if that doesn't give you any problems, then nightly if that's what the instructions tell you to do. If you're still experiencing a reaction, perhaps retinols aren't for you; step down to skincare with peptide technology. Always use retinol treatments at night, never in the morning, and shield with SPF; do NOT use them on holiday because retinol thins skin, decreasing its protective capacity, making it more vulnerable to sun damage and pigmentation. It can also become more sensitive. I often advise people to use retinol in winter for the most impressive results.

Q: Are doctors' skincare products stronger?

If you're seeing a dermatologist and they are giving you a prescription for a registered medical product, yes – but a doctor's range that you can buy online or in shops, no; it's almost certainly no different to everything else that's out there (unless they've done research and invented a new patented molecule). I'm always interested to check out whether skin doctors who put their names to ranges actually use them/sell them in their own clinics – because that shows they really believe in them.

Q: What is layering?

It's a way to get more active textures and ingredients into your skin. You apply consecutive products from thin to thick, for instance with a dry skin, you layer with serum/oil/cream. I liken it to eating out: a starter, a main course, a dessert.

Q: I have sensitive skin; I've bought loads of hypoallergenic products and they're not helping…

Hypoallergenic products can have long INCI (International Nomenclature Cosmetic Ingredients) lists that include fragrance-masking ingredients and preservatives. They may claim to be 'dermatologist-tested' but they're still complex products, with as many as 30 or 40 ingredients. Dial down; switch to fewer products, with fewer ingredients, and check out the advice for sensitive skin on p.44.

Q: Does exercising really age your face?

'Jogger's face' is a real phenomenon, common to those who do a lot of impact exercise. We're familiar with the way that jogging up and down can slacken the neck and bust area (hence the need for sports bras), but the same is also happening to your face; increased movement causes stretching of the facial tissues and eventually sagging. If you're outside running, you may also be picking up sun damage, too, breaking down the supportive fibres. Don't wear make-up when you exercise; always wear SPF; wash straight after sports to remove sweat from your face; introduce anti-slackening products into your regime. But why not consider switching to lower-impact exercise? Try cycling or fast walking to get an aerobic workout without too much bouncing up and down.

Q: Does swimming ruin your skin and hair?

Exposure to the chemicals and chlorine in pools can completely unbalance skin and hair. If you're swimming in those situations, put a few drops of oil or balm onto skin to protect it in the water. Work conditioner through your hair before you swim. Ozonically purified pools are kinder to skin, as is wild swimming. Get into the sea, if you can! People pay good money for thalassotherapy treatments to lie in a mineral-rich flotation tank, but you can get that for free if you swim in the sea.

Q: My face shape has changed – what can I do?

This is a normal part of the ageing process, but it is possible to firm the facial contours somewhat with electrical stimulation, either in salons or using at-home micro-current devices, which firm up the underlying muscles. Switch to firming products in your regime, but also learn make-up tricks to mimic the effects of a facelift (see p.170) – even putting your blusher on in a different place can work wonders. And why not change your hairstyle? Embrace the change. Show it off. It's going to happen to everyone.

Q: My products are rolling off my skin – what's happening?

It might be dead skin, as the result of not exfoliating properly, but it's more likely to be the firming or tightening agent in a product (mostly likely a serum) that is clashing with your other products and 'pilling', like a jumper does. If you're after a firming effect, you may want to buy a serum and moisturiser from within the same range, as these will have been tested together to ensure this doesn't happen. If you want to mix your ranges, use a thinner layer of your serum and wait until it's completely dry (maybe use the time to brush your teeth), before moisturising. Play with timings and quantity of product and you may find a workaround.

Q: What can I do about my pigmentation?

First off: shade is your friend. Hats. Trees. Umbrellas. SPF, of COURSE! But when it comes to treating pigmentation, you might want to focus on making improvements over the winter months with glycolics, retinols or vitamin C (see Ingredients matter p.127); it's much easier for the skin to recover and for pigmentation to diminish when it isn't being assaulted daily by UV light.

Q: What can I do about scars?

I used to work alongside the medical team at Grayshott Health Spa, helping amputees, mastectomy patients and those recovering from open heart surgery, so I'm very familiar with scars. And we all have them. Scarred skin is new, thin and very vulnerable, and it must be kept out of the sun for one to two years. As soon as you're given your doctor's go-ahead, make sure the scar gets plenty of moisture; water-based moisturising gels are ideal. I also recommend carrying vitamin E capsules with you when you're out and about; massage the contents of a vitamin E capsule into your scar very gently, several times a day. Be patient; scar treatment takes time, but it does work.

Acne scarring and pitting must also be treated with great gentleness. If it's fresh scarring, get into a regime of using a lightweight moisturiser and lightweight SPF. Much later, you can look at treatments like glycolics and laser treatments, but you need to wait until your acne has basically entirely disappeared before embarking on any of those. Blue light therapy is brilliant at calming down the angriness of spots and acne; you can now buy devices to do this at home.

Don't ever think that sunbeds and sunbathing can help with scars; these darken and thicken new skin of all tones. As a scar is new skin, you'll end up with a scar that's more visible than before.

Q: Can I mix ranges?

You can cherry pick, for sure, but don't choose products with the same active ingredients. You wouldn't eat the same for all three courses at a meal, would you? My rule is: the simpler your skincare regime, the easier it is to mix ranges. As your regime becomes more complex, there can be interactions. You could keep a beauty diary and when you slot something in, assess what happens to your skin over two or three skin cycles before introducing something else or switching. And remember: nobody needs two or three serums – you need one, otherwise you'll start to reach product overload and risk sensitivity (and overdraft!).

BAD BOTOX

Injectables have become so commonplace that there are now such things as Botox parties, held up and down the country and all over the world. There's a huge risk that something like this can go wrong; I've seen more than one drooping post-Botox brow, which means that person has to wait to return to normal over a period of months. It's just common sense that the results you'll get are likely to be very, very different from that A-list celebrity who can afford to travel to be treated by the best person in the world. I've seen lumps under the skin from filler that has hardened, or facelifts that have been done so tight the sides of the mouth have been stretched into a non-flattering grin. I urge you to try the other avenues in this book instead, and feel happy in your own skin!

A word about 'tweakments'

Everyone is different. Everyone is normal. So don't measure yourself against someone who makes a full-time job out of looking good...

Open any glossy magazine or turn on many TV shows and you'll be faced by countless images of 'perfection': glossy, polished and almost completely unattainable for most of us.

What's really important for us all to understand is that these individuals 'in the front line' of showbusiness or modelling go to enormous lengths to look good. If you add up the cost of the self-tanning, make-up artist, hair extensions, personal trainers, injections, 'tweakments', as well as the personal chefs, stylists etc, you will reach an annual total that is beyond most! When it's someone's job to look good, there are no lengths they won't go to, to keep looking their best. And you can pretty much guarantee that when they aren't in front of a camera or on a set, their time is almost entirely taken up by this other 'full-time job' – *getting ready* to be in front of the camera.

The trouble is, it sets the bar much too high for the rest of us. Normal people, who haven't got the budget or the time to embark on that hamster wheel of self-care. When I look at that high-maintenance individual, I rarely think: 'Gosh, you look fab.' I actually see insecurity. Why did they feel the need, particularly in the case of fillers or surgery, to go down that route? In the real world, there's no such thing as a straight nose or perfect boobs – so why would you feel so unhappy about a part of yourself that you'd undergo elective surgery, with all the risks that are attached to that? Is it really so important to be a size 8 that you need to start each day with a two-hour session with a personal trainer at 6 a.m., leaving the nanny to run the kids to school?

There's certainly a huge amount of pressure from the doctors and practitioners these celebrities engage with. 'We can make your face look more equal.' 'We can make your eyes less hooded.' They show a computer-generated image, and having made that person feel insecure about looking a certain way, they take advantage of that vulnerability. And as soon as you've had one thing done, you can lose sight of how you really look – and it's a slippery slope towards more fillers, more Botox, more surgery…

I have had negative comments on social media along the lines of 'Don't you think it's time you had some work done?', or 'Time for some Botox, Alison!' It happens to everyone in the public eye, at some point – and sure, it causes a wobble. But as I've woven throughout this book, there's so much that you can do to make the most of what you've got without going to that expense and risk.

I find it disappointing that few celebs will say they get work done (Dolly Parton is a rare exception!). It still takes guts to admit in Hollywood that anything but nature and good genes have played a part in how you look today. Even the owners of cosmetics brands may pretend their 'flawlessness' is all down to the products they're selling. I believe advice about beauty products should ONLY come from people who haven't had work done.

Let's also think of the next generation. If you, as a parent, have cosmetic surgery, fillers or expression-freezing jabs perpetuating this unrealistic ideal of 'perfection', you'll never be able to say 'No, you mustn't!', when your child asks for a boob job or to have their nose straightened.

So when friends ask me, 'Should I get X, Y or Z done?', I always say that there is no need. Because when I look at them, I see the *whole person*. When I look at any 'real' person – my friend, you, a sister, a son, a colleague – the most important things for me are your character, your honesty, your smile, your friendship, your talent, your intelligence. Those are the things that count so far as I'm concerned. That's what real beauty is. All this outer beauty stuff should help you to feel confident and happy in your own skin.

Wake up
to make-up

"

Make-up can enhance every face, at every stage of life

With modern textures and clever techniques, make-up can enhance every face, at every stage of life (and, if you like, nobody need even know it's there!). I always say to people that there's no need for surgery – you just need to know the right make-up tips!

I trained as a make-up artist during my early beauty training, and went on to train with legendary names like Ruby Hammer and Glauca Rossi. But what sets me apart is that I've never done red carpet, catwalk or editorial make-up; all my experience is on 'real' faces. What matters to me is helping people find looks that work in real life: the everyday work make-up, the brows that make you feel more confident when you're running out for a quick errand, the grab-and-run make-up for meeting friends.

My own first memories of make-up are crystal clear. Most days, my mum wore a tinted moisturiser and lipstick, but about twice a year, when we went out somewhere, it would be foundation with blusher, eyeshadow and lipstick (and her hair done, always). I remember the wonderful ritual of getting ready, and even now the sense of anticipation you get from prepping for a big night out or an event like a wedding is an important part of the experience itself, helping you get in the right mindset. It was my mum, by the way, who bought me my first make-up essentials: the pink-coloured concealer, the mascara and blue eyeliner that gave me the confidence to get out of the door and off to school.

I never listen to anyone if they tell me that make-up is somehow frivolous or unimportant: try telling that to someone who's just been at a Look Good, Feel Better workshop that offers make-up and grooming sessions for cancer patients. Everyone taking part comes out with their confidence transformed – often into the arms of a partner, with both of them in tears, because they look and feel like themselves again. 'I've got my wife back,' is a comment that the professionals hear. I've worked with people undergoing cancer treatment, and I can tell you:

for someone who's lost their brows or lashes, or whose skin has gone haywire because of chemo, make-up is nothing less than magic.

If you're ill or feeling down, make-up can put a new face on you – and on life itself. You can use make-up to make you look well again, and to hide the effects of a bad night. It can disguise features you don't love and (importantly) play up your good bits.

In the past few years, make-up technology has made incredible advances, for example, natural and 'free-from' lines have been revolutionised, with textures rivalling mainstream choices. And it's not just a women's thing now: there are great men's make-up ranges and make-up bars, so guys can take advantage of make-up's confidence-boosting power. (You know when Chanel launch a range of make-up for men that the world's changing, thank goodness.)

Today's make-up technology means that alongside the 'fashion' colours and products which are fun to play with, there are so, so many options that deliver seamless results, so that you look like you – but just that bit more vibrant. So: whether you want a totally natural, can't-tell-it's-there-look or the equivalent of make-up 'surgery', I'm about to share my best secrets with you. Remember, though, the best make-up starts with the best skin care (see the Skin section for more).

> **If you're ill or feeling down, make-up can put a new face on you — and on life itself.**

The make-up toybox

Make-up should be fun! And there's lots of fun to be had simply playing around with your existing products to achieve new looks.

Schedule time to assess what you already own, to practise a new look, master the art of liquid liner or perfect your Christmas party make-up. (Better now than at the last minute, with a taxi ticking outside or with someone drumming their fingers impatiently.)

- **Set aside part of a day or an evening.**

To be honest, daytime is better because of the light; a summer's evening is fine but you do need daylight to see how products truly look on your skin. Alternatively, buy a daylight bulb for one of your table lamps. Ideally, you also want a decent-sized mirror that stands up on its own, rather than a hand mirror; you might want to upgrade your mirror to one with built-in daylight/night light options. Sit facing the light source so it strikes both sides of your face evenly.

The best time in the diary for this is the seasonal change over, twice a year – if you're getting out your jumpers and thick tights, you need to adjust your make-up too: out with the shimmer and glow, in with the velvets and mattes.

Pour yourself a glass of wine, make a cup of tea, or enjoy a cool glass of water. This is real 'me-time', so make the most of it.

- **Step 1: Lay out your kit.**

If you have a dressing table, that's perfect; if not, a table (perhaps a dining table) where you can line everything up. Put a towel down to stop things rolling away. Get out everything from everywhere you stash make-up; every last drawer or box.

- **Step 2: Group your products.**

Zone things: like with like.

- **Step 3: You'll probably have to say 'goodbye' to some things…**
What you're trying to do is pull together a core make-up bag of essentials. Old mascaras and lipsticks should go: there is the potential for bacteria to breed and spread infection to eyes. The oils in lipsticks can go rancid, or change colour. Powder textures and most pencils have a long shelf-life, so should be ok, but you might need to sharpen.

- **Step 4: Wash your brushes.**
Brushes should be washed at least once a week; if you've got spotty skin, wash them each time you use them. You can buy brush cleaners, spritzes, spinning brush-clean gizmos, but they're all alcohol- and chemical-based and personally, as someone who suffers from eczema, the ingredients can sensitise my skin. I use my face wash or a gentle shampoo. Don't submerge brushes beyond the point where the handle joins the metal shank; that's where the glue is, and it may dissolve. Dry them with the bristles hanging over the edge of the surface they're resting on, so the air can circulate. (A towel can help stop them rolling off here, too). Thoroughly wash any sponges/beauty blenders, too.

- **Step 5: Clean everything that's left.**
Wash and dry any bags and boxes you keep your stash in. Using cotton pads soaked in micellar water or spritzed with hand sanitiser, wipe around lids, clean the tops of compacts. Use a little squirt of glass cleaner and some kitchen towel to clean mirrors. Use a hairdryer on pots of balm or balm-style blushers, to melt the formula and reform them to a smooth finish.

- **Step 6: Put together different kits.**
This is a bit more fun! Assemble a kit for everyday use. Maybe one for your desk, if you've got 'extras', or for the hall mirror. See if you can create an edit of just five or six products in each bag, as this is probably all that you really need for everyday.

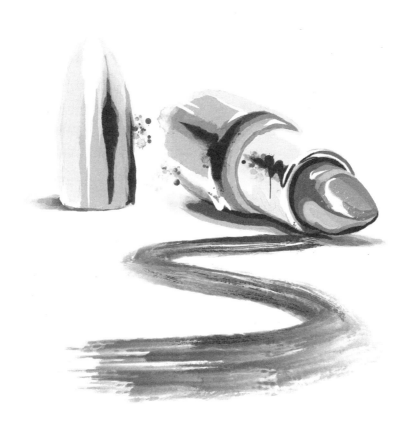

I don't recommend a full kit for the car, because the temperatures outside can be too extreme for cream textures and pencils. The easiest car kit is an all-in-one foundation powder and a tinted lip gloss. Think about assembling a kit for holidays and one with your evening make-up, too.

Alison's Tip

Work on your technique. Most of us are really good at applying, say, eyeliner to one eye, but not so good with the other. This is the perfect time to practise. Maybe tune into some YouTube video tutorials (perhaps my channel!) where you can see different techniques demoed, to watch and learn. This is ideal if you have an important event ahead; use this time as a rehearsal.

Ace of bases

Foundation technology has been revolutionised over the past decade, offering seamless, can't-tell-it-from-real-skin results. Here's how to find your perfect finish and complexion match…

Most foundation brands now offer an incredibly wide shade spectrum, to match every skin tone under the sun – a definite sign that the beauty world is changing for the better. More good news: if you're on a budget, it's great to know that the high street now has a fantastic foundation offering, as state-of-the-art technologies have trickled down to the mainstream.

Nevertheless, staring at a foundation fixture in a store can be completely overwhelming. First and foremost, it's about problem-solving, to find the best choice to enhance your skin. Most of us still need a wardrobe of complexion finishes: one for weekends, for holidays/summer, for work and for special occasions…

HAVE FUN EXPERIMENTING

Looking at the make-up you have, play around with some items you haven't used for a while and see what new effects you can create, without having to buy anything new.

1. Try upgrading your foundation application from fingers to a synthetic brush; this can give a more polished look.

2. Try using a very large brush with your powder, to see if it gives a more diffused glow.

3. Do you have a scarily strong-toned lipstick that you don't use? Try it over balm as a sheer stain. Try also applying it with a lip brush: you'll get two completely different looks.

4. Dip a fine brush into micellar water, then into dark-toned eye shadow to see if it works as a liner, too (p.s. you should never spit on brushes to dampen them!).

5. Try lip colours on cheeks, too, and in the eye socket for a super-quick, pulled-together, all-in-one look.

FIRST, CHOOSE YOUR TEXTURE...

Before you get to shade selection, you need to choose the right texture for your skin type and your desired level of coverage and finish. If you have normal skin, you can use any texture you like, but if not, choosing the right make-up for your complexion type will give performance that will last all day (and/or evening). For oilier or combination skin, choose mattifying or 'velvet' textures. Normal-to-dry skins choose moisturising or serum formulas. (Hyaluronic acid can also be added to your chosen complexion cover product to loosen the texture, perhaps for a more casual look.)

Tinted moisturiser

Best for: All skins

Quick and easy, the clue's in the name: these are moisturising creams with a slight tint, offering lightweight, barely there coverage that simply evens out skin tones. Some of them feature luminising particles to add a whisper of glow as well as a touch of colour. Just as you can find oil-free moisturisers, there are oil-free tinted moisturisers for oily and combination skins and these are now available in a range of shades, rather than the old one-shade-suits-all options. For a lot of people, a tinted moisturiser is a great 'weekend' or 'holiday' foundation choice.

Alphabet creams

Best for: All skins

These originated in Korea and are lighter than typical foundations; great for young or problem-free skins, instead of foundation. For more mature skins, they're used in the same way as primers.

BB creams are short for 'Beauty Balms', and are similar to a tinted moisturiser, often with quite a lot of radiance in the formula.

'CC' stands for 'Colour Control' or 'Colour Correcting', and these lightweight creams feature blurring pigments to even out skin tone, particularly redness or discolouration. For a while there were also DD creams, but these have pretty much come and gone. And if you're wondering, these are all terms dreamed up by marketing departments.

The coverage and finish varies massively both in BB and CC creams. As with any foundation, you really need to try these on your skin before buying, as some offer a lot of concealment and others, none at all. Because of all the variables, try before you buy.

Liquid foundation

Best for: All skins

These range from ultra-sheer to velvety finishes, and are 'buildable' to get greater depth of coverage with a foundation brush or beauty blender. Foundation technology means that even thin liquid foundations now offer fantastic, full coverage.

Oil-free options are available for oilier/combination complexions, which may be water-based or clay-based to absorb shine. Others have hydrating benefits, ideal for normal to dry complexions; the drier your skin, the richer the texture you need in a foundation.

If you're not buying from a beauty counter with an assistant who can run you through different finishes and skin type suitability, do your research online: the name of the product is often a good clue to how it appears on the skin – 'radiant', 'glow', 'velvet' or 'matte'.

For ease of use, opt for a pump rather than a bottle that you need to pour the foundation out of, which can get messy. I've had experience with faulty pumps – if that happens to you, don't hesitate to take the product back to the store you bought it from, or return it to a website. (It's always good to keep mail order returns forms somewhere safe, rather than throwing them away.)

Don't dot liquid foundation straight onto the face; apply a few drops to the back of your (freshly-washed) hand or a metal lid, then use a foundation brush to pick up the formula and apply to your face.

Cream foundation

Best for: Dry skin

The drier your complexion, the richer your foundation should be – buttery, nourishing and moisturising. Apply cream foundation by picking up the

PRIMER: UNDERWEAR FOR YOUR FOUNDATION

Primers have revolutionised make-up. They are applied as an extra layer, after your skincare and before foundation, and perform a couple of tricks: they smooth out the surface and blur imperfections, and allow make-up to be applied more smoothly. They also turbo-charge the staying power of make-up. If you haven't ever used a primer, do, do, DO – they're a revelation, especially before a special event.

You choose your primer depending on the finish you want. There are **glow/luminising primers**, for skin to look radiant and lit-from-within. There are **mattifying primers**, ideal for oily skins (if you have combination skin or menopause skin, apply a mattifying primer to shine-prone areas only). Then there are **line-smoothing primers** which even out the skin's surface.

You can also buy **colour-correcting primers**, which appear lilac, apricot, pink, green or yellow in the tube/bottle, but smoothed onto skin work to correct skin tone. Once upon a time, these only came in green, and were so opaque they basically made you look like Shrek, but they have improved so much. Here are some options:

- **Green** tones down redness/rosacea/acne.
- **Yellow** is great if you have blue veins under the surface, especially around the eyes, and for adding warmth to a dark complexion.
- **Lavender** counterbalances yellowness in fair skins, to make skin more glowy.
- **Pink** adds a healthy, rosy glow to washed-out skin.
- **Peach/apricot** is good for hiding dark circles, age spots and areas of pigmentation.

If you have a problem with eye make-up creasing or lipstick disappearing/bleeding, you might want to step up to a dedicated 'zoned' primer for the lips and/or eyes, some of which also offer skincare benefits.

cream with a brush, wiping on the edge of the jar, and smoothing into skin. Or use the back-of-the-hand technique as for a liquid foundation, above.

Stick foundation
Best for: Normal/dry

Definitely the easiest to use: a swivel-up thick stick that can be used as concealer/foundation – you literally dot and stripe it over moisturised skin and blend with a brush or fingers – ideal if you're in a hurry. Or try applying with a dampened beauty blender for a subtler finish. Because there's no risk of spillage, throw into your bag for touch-ups, later on.

Mineral foundation
Best for: All skins /sensitive/spot-prone

These can be great for oily skins, breakouts and sensitive complexions because they don't have oils, emulsifiers and preservatives (they're inert powders, so none are required), and don't clog pores. The zinc in mineral foundation is a great ingredient for spotty skins.

You can build mineral foundation to a full finish, using a kabuki brush (see pp.162–63) that you swirl onto skin. But oh, there's real potential for mess: these are best for home use because the powder can get everywhere if the lid comes off. So don't carry your mineral foundation around with you; there will come a day when you open up your make-up bag and it looks like Pompeii in there. Some mineral make-up brands now offer convenient compacts featuring pressed mineral foundations to get round this problem, which are also swirled onto skin until you reach your desired level of coverage.

Cream compact foundation
Best for: Normal/dry

Applied with a puff or a sponge for buildable coverage, these have a cream texture and may offer skincare benefits. Compact foundations are great for on-the-go touch-ups, are spill-proof, and ideal if you like to put your make-up on during your morning commute by public transport. They can work out more expensive as they don't last as long as creams or sticks.

Powder compact/all-in-one foundation
Best for: Oily/combination/normal

Applied with a puff or a brush, these can also double as a face-finishing powder over a cream or liquid foundation. These are technically suitable for all skin types but may not be comfortable on a very dry skin. Again, super-portable. If you like a compact foundation, play around with brushes to get a range of finishes. A small brush will give a denser coverage, while a large, fluffy brush delivers a lighter, airier finish. You can use the same product with a small, flat brush (i.e. an eyeshadow brush) to cover a spot or even out the colour on your eyelids.

NOW, CHOOSE YOUR SHADE...

The good news here is that the shade range for foundations has increased massively. Textures are now so seamless (thanks to self-levelling, adjusting pigments) that they are also far more forgiving if you do choose one that's a shade or two too light or dark. If you're shopping in store, ask about a money-back guarantee if the shade doesn't turn out to be right (or check the returns policy of a website). On a TV shopping channel, you may get up to a 60-day no-questions-asked refund. Here are my top tips for choosing the right shade for you:

- **Try foundation on the side of your face, on the jawline.**
  In general, foundation needs to blend seamlessly with the shade of your skin under your cheek, at jaw level. However, foundation doesn't *have* to match your natural skin tone perfectly. These days, many brands offer shades with cool, neutral and warm undertones, and going for a shade slightly warmer than your natural complexion

can be very flattering. Just remember to also bring up the colour on your neck (see tip below).

- **Always check a foundation shade in daylight.**
Not doing this is the No.1 fast track to making a foundation mistake, because you can't check the colour match properly in artificial light. Shop during daytime if you can, and carry a small compact mirror and go outside the store to look at the shade/s on your jawline in natural light.

- **If you can't get to a store, check out 'virtual try-on technology'.**
Expect to see more and more websites offering 'try-on' virtual shade finders, where you take a selfie and the website or app technology suggests a match. Alternatively, some brands have developed genius questionnaires which take you step-by-step through finding your right shade – and they're surprisingly accurate.

Alison's Tip

If there's a contrast between the colour of your face and neck (which can be paler), I've several tricks you can try:

- Use a bronzer on the neck, to bring the colour up.

- Use a gradual self-tanner or add a couple of tanning drops to your night cream, to do the same.

- Buy a specific long-wear foundation, designed not to budge, and take it down the neck.

Choosing brushes

There are so many brushes and sponges out there – what does what, and which do you really need?

1. **A foundation brush**
   Will give you a fuller, more perfect finish, allowing you to build up layer by layer.

2. **A concealer brush**
   Normally smaller and flatter for precision application.

3. **A beauty blender**
   Generally egg-shaped beauty sponges, these take you from medium to full coverage. Used damp they're great for getting a smooth finish. Both beauty blenders and sponges also let you get right under the eye.

4. **A sponge**
   Allows you to build up fine layers of foundation very delicately, when used fairly wet. Use just slightly damp for a fuller coverage.

5. **A kabuki brush**
   A domed brush for using to swirl on mineral powder make-up.

6. **A powder brush**
   For applying bronzers and highlighters, you can use a big, fluffy dome brush, but I prefer a fan-shaped brush. The fan is great for building fine layers and gives a lighter, more featherweight and natural-looking finish. (Also see p.173 for my favourite blusher brush.)

7. **Your fingers**
   Any foundation (except powder) can be applied with fingers for speed, or if you really like an ultra-natural finish. But you can take off almost as much as you put on, if you're not careful.

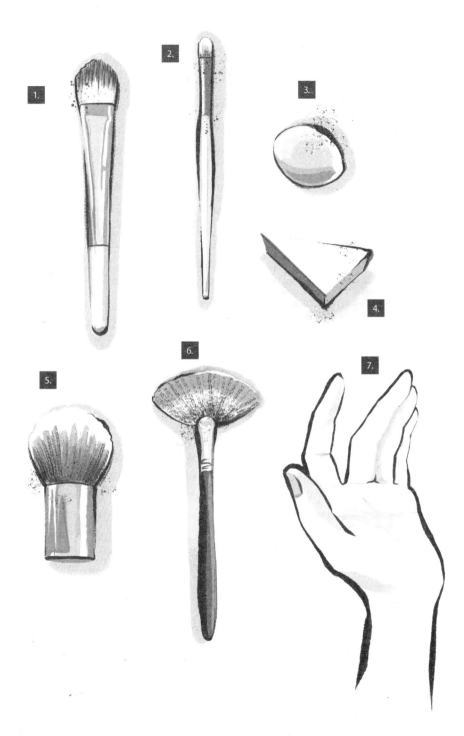

How to apply foundation

Your step-by-step to the perfect, flawless base...

1   If you're applying powder foundation, concealer goes on first (see opposite). If you're applying liquid foundation, concealer goes on after.

2   For a light finish, put a couple of drops onto your fingertips and smooth into skin as if you were using a tinted moisturiser.

3   For more coverage, brush the foundation onto your face in a downward direction, so the brush goes over the pores and doesn't sink into them. Apply first to areas that need most coverage, and blend over areas that need evening out.

4   Once applied, press your fingers onto the skin to warm the foundation or gently bounce a damp beauty blender over the skin; this helps the foundation sink in and allows the colour to merge with your own skin.

5   Brows always pick up a bit of foundation when you're using a brush, so clean up the brow area with a cotton bud to get back to your natural brow shade.

6   If you're using liquid/cream foundation, finish with the lightest sweep of face powder in your chosen finish, applied with a powder brush – matte, velvety, luminous; it's your choice and there are powders that deliver all those finishes and more. There are now even hydrating powders that offer a non-drying finish. This will 'set' make-up to ensure it stays put for longer. I prefer a 'fan brush' (see p.162 as this gives a super-light finish). And if you do use powder, apply it on the face in a downward direction to avoid it making pores more obvious.

Alison's Tip

A double-ended foundation brush can be useful, with a smaller brush on the other end that makes it easy to get close to the lash-line and apply to lids.

The art of concealment

Concealers come in two types. Many of us need both…

- **Coverage concealers**

These are for red veins, dark spots, spots and dark circles. Just a few years ago it would have been unthinkable to find a make-up brand with as many as 30 shades of concealer, but now that's not unusual. Coverage concealers should therefore always be skin-matched (same advice as for foundations, see p.160).

Concealers are generally patted into skin to build coverage till you reach the level you want, which tends to be matte or velvety. If you've great skin, or want a light finish, sometimes a dab of concealer can be enough to even out skin tone, without needing foundation.

- **Light-reflecting concealers**

These disguise dark circles, shadows and fine lines and wrinkles (such as the furrow lines between the brows or the fold from nose to the corners of the mouth). There are fewer shade options because they're much easier on the skin tone; they bring freshness, lightness and brightness to the face.

Concealer how-to

There are six 'levels' of concealer application, ranging from light everyday coverage through concealing dark circles, right through to hiding all darkness, sunken areas and droopiness.

Level 1 For a light finish (also suitable for men) you can use a normal or illuminating concealer. Apply inside the inner corner of the eye and just under the inner corner where shadows tend to be blueish on almost everyone. Tap with fingers to press into skin, for a fresh, invisible finish.

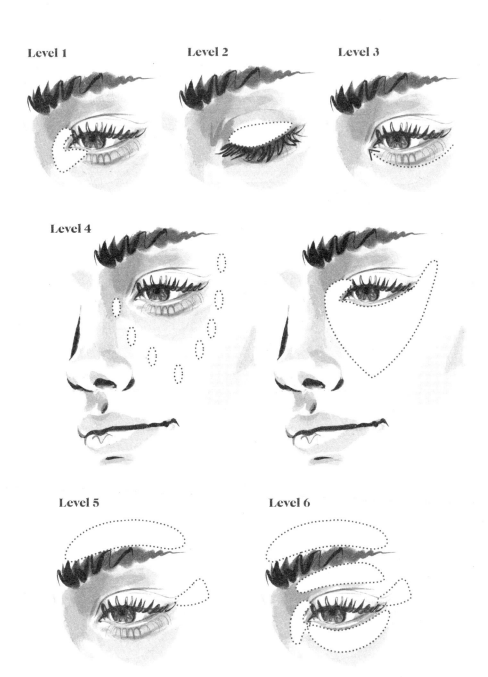

Six levels of concealer application, from light to full coverage

Level 2 To brighten and 'lift' the eye, apply your concealer above the lid area, not below. You can do this with a liquid or pot concealer or with a stick or regular foundation. This distracts from any under-eye circles, like a magic trick. Use a concealer brush and blend/press into skin with fingers.

Level 3 This is where you take the concealer, using a concealer brush, in a semi-circle under the eye from the outer corner to the inner corner. The inner corner is darker, so blend inwards. This will ensure more product is deposited where you need it, on the darkest area. Press into skin with fingers.

Level 4 This is for a sunken socket or a 'ridged' under-eye area, usually as a result of significant puffiness – or exhaustion! Apply dots of concealer in a V-shape under the eye using the brush or wand from the product. With a sponge, using a tapping movement, blend the concealer into your foundation from the outer edge towards the inner corner of the eye/nose bone and also along the cheekbone, where it acts as a highlighter. I then like to switch to a concealer brush to get better access to this area and underneath the lower lash-line, blending as I go. Press into skin with fingers.

Level 5 This is where you build on Level 4 to also add a lighter concealer above the brow, which works to 'lift' the whole eye area. Also focus on applying to the outer corner of the eye, in an upwards direction. Lots of us have blue shadows here too and it also counteracts age-related droopiness. Press into skin with fingers, without disturbing the concealer.

Level 6 Add extra light reflection with a luminising/highlighting concealer on the fuller coverage areas and high points. It gives a fresh finish and can actually disguise heavier coverage.

INVISIBLE MAKE-UP

With a few products and tricks, you can create such a subtle look that nobody will know you're wearing make-up, yet it can still be polished enough to make you feel pulled together and confident. Great for guys, no make-up-wearers, or anyone, on low-key days. Here are my tips for 'invisible' make up:

- **Add a few tanning drops to your moisturiser.** Or use a daily facial self-tanner. Everyone will be able to see your natural complexion, but it will have a little extra warmth.

- **Use a CC cream.** See p.156 for more on these, but they're brilliant for just evening out your skin without looking like you're wearing foundation.

- **Have your brows and/or lashes tinted.** If you're fair or grey-haired this can make a huge, instant difference.

- **Try a mascara that gradually adds a tint to lashes.** Day by day, you'll get a little extra colour.

- **Use 'clear' make-up formulas.** You can get clear mascaras (great for dark lashes) and brow gels for a groomed finish. Clear blotting powders and balms can be used either on naked skin or over make-up, for a conditioned, natural-looking glow.

- **Add a touch of liquid blusher or a skin tint to cheeks.** These are see-through formulas to add undetectable, natural-looking colour to lips and cheeks.

Blushing beauty

Children don't need blusher – they have a natural, rosy glow which looks fresh. But as we age, skin becomes more washed out, so we can use blusher to mimic that – and on some days, it can make us look human again!

Blushers come in an increasingly wide choice of textures, from gels and tints to balms and powders. They can be used on their own or you can layer them for different textures and longer wear.

Gel/liquid blusher

For a sheer, realistic flush, dab onto cheeks with a finger or a doe-foot applicator. These products are good on bare skin, rather than over foundation. You've only got about 10–20 seconds of application time before they 'set', so do one cheek at a time and blend, before the opposite cheek. Good for a sporty or natural look or as the base layer to a powder blusher.

Cream blusher

Easy to use, and ideal for touching up on-the-go later in the day. Can be used over moisturised bare skin or over foundation. For best and most long-lasting results, apply with a synthetic brush. For long-wear, 'set' the blusher with a layer of powder blusher or face powder.

Powder blusher

The longest-lasting style of blusher, apply with a brush and over foundation, or it will go on patchy and won't last. High-quality powder blushers often have silky textures that deliver a sheer, seamless, buildable finish without the hard edges they used to be known for.

BLUSHER MASTERCLASS

I am often asked about how to apply blusher – and where on the face is best. And in fact, that changes as we age, so here's my blusher-through-the-stages-of-life tutorial.

You will need a full, angled brush (see p.173). Blusher goes on after foundation, concealer and face-shaping (contour) products, or it can be your best friend for a quick look just on top of tinted moisturiser.

- **Blusher for younger faces**

Sweep the blusher from the centre of the cheek to the hairline, in line with the top of the ear. For as long as you still have firm cheekbone contours, you can keep following this angle.

- **'Facelift' blusher**

As we age, blush generally needs to be applied differently. Angle the sweep of your blusher brush from the middle of the cheek (no further in than in line with the pupil of the eye) towards the middle of your ear. You're leaving a bigger gap above the cheek than with the younger-face blusher, and almost filling in a 'triangle' of skin below the cheekbone, because the contours have drooped. Fluff and blend as you go.

- **Natural/apple-cheeked blusher**

This is a fresh-faced look, to be worn with natural, everyday make-up (it wouldn't go with a smoky eye). Smile to find your cheek's 'apple'. Use a blusher gel, applied with a beauty blender sponge (or fingers), stippling it onto the centre of the cheeks and blending outwards for a rounded look that is glowy and unstructured.

- **Add some glow...**

Add a 'low-glow' highlighter powder above the cheekbones, applied with an angled blusher brush (see p.73). Work outwards towards the ears above your blusher, to create the illusion of a wider and higher space. You can also sweep your brush down the bone of the nose from just between the eyebrows and just above and below the brows.

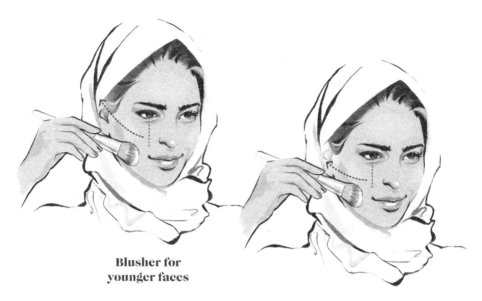

Blusher for younger faces

'Facelift' blusher

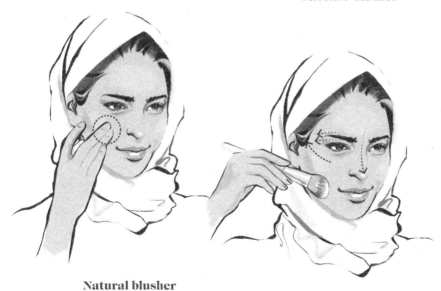

Natural blusher

Add some glow

Blusher masterclass: where to apply your blusher and highlighter

- **Long-wear blusher**
If you have a big day or night ahead, you might want to apply gel or cream blusher first, and then layer on powder blusher.

Alison's tip ———————————————————

Do your blusher after your foundation and brows. Sometimes that can be such a 'wow' that you can get away with less eye-work and a subtler lipstick. Mix it up sometimes and try changing the order of your application.

AND THE PERFECT SHADE...

When it comes to the ideal shade of blusher, take the cue from your clothes and the warmth of your skin tone: for every shade of blusher, there's a warmer and a cooler version. Which colours in your wardrobe make your eyes look brighter and your complexion fresher – pinks, or corals or other 'warm' tones? If you wear a lot of brown and have a cooler, more blue-toned skin tone, meanwhile, a browny pink can be really flattering. You can always add a 'pop' – just the lightest whisper – of a fashion shade of blush, over your regular shade. This is something to experiment with when you're at the make-up toybox, see p.151.

Alison's Tip ———————————————————

Next time you come back from a brisk walk, have a look in the mirror. Your most flattering blusher shade will be similar to that natural flush on your cheeks. Take a selfie and look for a blusher that recreates that shade!

There's no excuse for using animal hair brushes. The textures of today's synthetic brushes are finer and softer than natural hair make-up brushes ever were. My favourite blusher brush is the angled brush here.

If you need a brush for touching up blusher when out and about, buy a retractable or short-handled brush to avoid the bristles being bent out of shape because your brush is squished in your bag. If you're using powder blusher, you can load a little powder onto your retractable brush for a late-in-the-day touch-up, and you needn't carry the blusher itself. Alternatively, you can top up your cheeks with a little lipstick, applied and blended with fingertips.

BRONZERS

Bronzers aren't just about tanning; they are fantastic for perking up your skin tone and making you look healthy anytime – on holiday, post-illness, when you're tired etc. They're also an easy way to adjust your foundation shade to complement a new hair colour or a brightly coloured dress, taking it a little warmer. Everyone, whatever their skin tone, can benefit from a warming shade of bronzer.

For day-to-day, always use matte bronzer, not shimmer. There are now many different shades of bronzer available, a huge improvement on early bronzers with one, very orange shade. Nowadays, if a brand offers a single shade of bronzer and it's not right for you, head instead for a make-up artist brand, who'll offer a whole spectrum of bronzers with different undertones and shades for all skin tones.

- **For a quick, grab-and-run make-up.**
Use a big fluffy brush that you keep exclusively for bronzer. Apply matte bronzer around the 'circle of light', literally a circle around the outside of the face from hairline to under the cheekbones, the jaw and down the neck – the idea is that this, by omission, highlights the centre of the face. When you've done that and there's very little bronzer left on the brush, buff the centre of the face. This 'framing' with the bronzer will draw attention to eyes and lips.

- **Use a bronzer on the neck to even up skin tone.**
Apply matte bronzer down the neckline and to the collar/V of your shirt/jumper, rather than applying foundation. Bronzer can also be used to cover up pale sunglasses/ski goggles 'circles', or for evening up skin tone quickly if you've been wearing a mask. I also always keep bronzer handy for feet, when you want to wear sandals, post winter!

- **Face contouring.**
Sweep matte bronzer around the top of the forehead at the hairline, under the cheekbones and under the jawline. By omission this highlights the areas of the face you want to appear lifted.

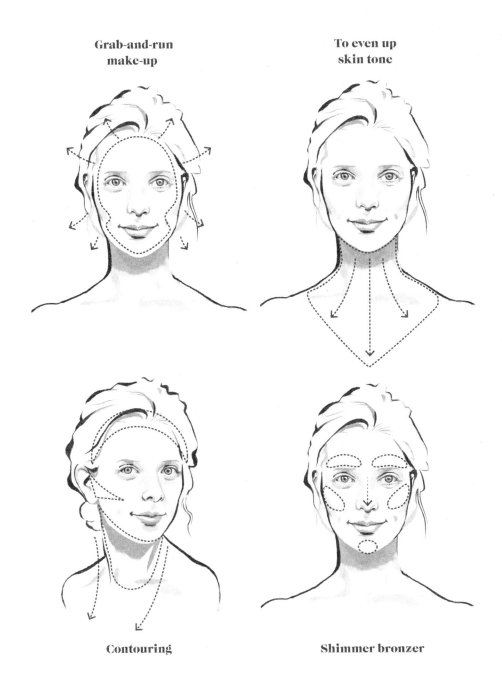

Grab-and-run make-up

To even up skin tone

Contouring

Shimmer bronzer

Bronzers: where to apply matte and shimmer bronzer

You can also add 'strobing', using a highlighter to further lift the cheekbones, brow bones and the upper jawline.

- **Shimmer bronzers are fun, but they're not for every day.** You want bronzer to look ultra-natural; shimmer bronzers do draw attention to the fact you're wearing make-up, because of the glimmer, so they're great on holiday or in summer, or for a glowy evening look, perhaps. Sweep onto the face where the sun naturally strikes: forehead, cheekbones and chin, with maybe a light sweep down the nose. Shimmer bronzers can also be used on the body, to accent body parts, swept across décolletage, shoulders, arms and down the shins and feet.

INSTANT GLOW MAKE-UP

This is my low-key, going to the supermarket, 'day off' look when I still want to be fresh-faced and glowy. If you want to wear make-up when at the gym or dance class, rather than removing it beforehand, this look will work for that, too.

1. Either choose a BB or tinted moisturiser, or add a couple of glow drops or drops of serum to your foundation or tinted moisturiser, for lighter coverage. Apply the foundation with fingertips in a downwards movement over the face, for a soft-not-so-heavy finish.

2. Use a big, fat, fluffy blending brush to blend your foundation, buffing in a downward direction.

3. If you'd like to even out your complexion a little more, use a luminising concealer on the inside corner of the eyes, the centre of the under-eyes and the lids, blending well. You can also blend this concealer into nose-to-mouth lines and frown lines between the brows.

4. Press your hands onto your face, lifting and repeating, warming the make-up into your skin so that it 'takes'.

5. **Grab-and-run brow** (see p.196), using a simple brow mascara or powder.

6. **Eyeliner Look 1** (see p.204).

7. Apply a blusher or a bronzer to your cheeks. Smile, so you can see the apples of the cheeks, and buff the blusher into cheeks and outwards towards hairline.

8. Dab your finger in the blusher or bronzer and use it to shade your outer eyelids. Add a touch of the powder to your lips and blend with your finger.

9. Add lip balm or gloss over the powder on your lips.

10. Apply mascara to upper lashes first, then lower lashes, when there's less product left on the wand.

11. If skin seems too glowy (if it's hot, for instance), finish with a touch of powder.

12. If you still feel you need a little more structure, squeeze the brush to create a narrower tip and apply more of the blusher/bronzer to your socket line.

Bronzers are fantastic for perking up your skin tone and making you look healthy anytime.

Lip tips

The skin on your lips is one of the most sensitive areas of your body, so let's look at how to care for this fragile area. Swiping on lip colour is the quickest way to change how you look. Is it any wonder we're lip-obsessed…?

THE BALMY ARMY

Slicking on a lip balm is one of the most instantly comforting beauty gestures we can make. The lip area is different to the skin anywhere else on your body, which is why it needs extra (and more regular) care. The cells are thin, flat, producing no oil or moisture of their own, so they lose water really quickly. If you're in any doubt, eat crisps when you've dry lips; that stinging feeling is a clue that lips are over-dry, and even cracked.

Being an outdoorsy type, lip balms are a must for me. I use them regularly, but not 'all the time', addictively. If you find yourself reapplying every hour or more, then your lip balm itself isn't moisturising enough and it's time to trade up. A good lip balm is a blend of nourishing oils, perhaps shea or cocoa butter, solidified with beeswax or candelilla wax. Lip balms can now also be anti-ageing treatment products, with higher price tags attached. If you are concerned about lip ageing, seek out a balm featuring an ingredient called MaxiLip, a clinically proven ingredient which is both plumping and works to treat wrinkles; press one of these balm or lip treatments into lips after application, and you can visibly see your lips plump slightly.

So far as I'm concerned, you can't have too many lip balms in your life, because lips dry out so much quicker than your face. I have them scattered around the house, next to the bed, next to the TV remote control, in the car. One of my best tips is to keep one by your toothbrush; toothpaste is incredibly drying, so slicking on a balm after brushing your teeth can be really soothing. Every now and then, because balms do somehow go walkabout, I'll round up the strays and slip one into a pocket of each jacket or coat, for outdoor lip protection. And men need lip balm, too! It's often a revelation when a chap tries one on his chapped lips. Here are some lip balm tips:

- Tinted lip balms are great for adding a hint of low-key colour for a no-make-up look, but I find the untinted balms to be better treatment products.

- Lip balm is often the first requirement for a child, after sunscreen. Try not to share them between family members, though, because of cross-contamination (see below).

- Be aware the demarcation line between the lips and your face is an area of particular sensitivity. When it's out of whack, you can get a red, flaky irritation line or even crustiness/soreness at the corners from yeast or stubborn fungal infections. The lip area is a common problem area for dermatitis or eczema. If your lips have gone beyond general dryness, try Blistex (which is medicated), or better still, ask a pharmacist for advice and/or a treatment.

- If you are prone to cold sores, definitely seek out a prescription formula from a doctor or pharmacist. If you get a cold sore, throw away any lip balms you may have used recently, to avoid contamination.

FEELING THE LIPSTICK LOVE

Doesn't everyone love lipstick…? It is the make-up item that can make the quickest, biggest difference to your appearance – literally in a flash. It can change the appearance of your skin tone and emphasise the colour of your eyes. The right lipstick is also a contrast against the white of your teeth and the whites of your eyes.

Lipstick can be your saving grace if you've run out of time for other make-up. A naked eye is no worry if you put a strong lipstick on – nobody will know you've overslept; they'll just admire your style! Dark glasses,

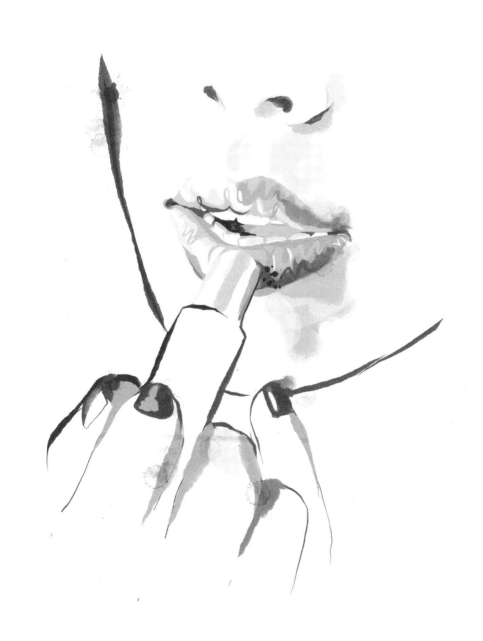

a baseball cap and a strong lip get me from country to town, double-quick. And for me, lipstick is an essential travel look, a chance to wear a different shade to what I'd wear at home, just as you might choose a different perfume to wear.

Here is a run-down of the different types out there:

Lip gloss

The textures and formulations of these have moved on apace since their sticky debut; if you abandoned them because your hair kept getting glued to your lips, glosses are worth revisiting. Offering sheer, shiny coverage, there are now longer-lasting glosses, but it's all relative because the more moisturising and glossy a lip formula is, the faster it will disappear. They're very versatile: use them over lipstick as a final glamorous sweep, or on bare lips for a subtle make-up look. They can even be pressed into cheekbones for a glossy highlighter.

Lip ink

These 'stain' colour onto the lips and are super long-lasting, applied with the built-in applicator. They can look scary in the tube but the secret is to apply lightly and blend with a finger, rather than an intense coat all over. They're great for something like a Zoom call or under a mask because the stain will stay put for hours. (These are also sometimes called LIP STAINS.) They can feel a little drying; you could apply over or under a balm, but be aware that this will shorten the time the ink stains your lips.

Lip oil

Supposedly a treatment product, because they have 'nourishing' ingredients (mango butter, jojoba, coconut) – but I have my doubts about that because there are no absorbent cells or pores on the lips for them to sink into. My experience is lip oils sit on the lip surface or even slide off. (Balms are thicker, and include ingredients like beeswax which make them stay put, acting as a barrier.) If you like the glossy finish, great – or the tint (some of these offer a sheer wash of colour) – but don't expect lip oils to stay put on the lips for long or help with dryness.

Lip velvet

Rich, highly pigmented liquid lipsticks. These are usually applied from a tube with an applicator. As with lip inks, you can go lightly and blend by tapping into lips with a finger rather than opt for the full-glamour, all-over velvet effect.

Matte lipstick

Tends to be longer-lasting than moisturising lipstick, delivering a matte finish – great if you want a high drama statement look, but be aware the matteness isn't always flattering on a more mature face, where a touch of shine will be more welcome.

Moisturising lipstick

Very popular lip make-up choices, with nourishing, plumping qualities and a high comfort factor. The downside: they'll probably need more frequent reapplication, the more moisturising your chosen formula is.

Alison's Tip

Less can be more! If you have a wardrobe of lipsticks you never wear, have a try-on session and edit them down (with eye make-up remover handy for taking off the lipsticks after trying each of them on). Some people have dozens of lipsticks in the same shade; all that's happening is they're cluttering your make-up kit. If you do have a wide shade range, try layering different shades on top of each other to see if there's a flattering new combination you can come up with, for an absolutely 'free' new look. You can use a hairdryer to melt them together in a pot.

CHOOSING THE RIGHT SHADE

How do you find your 'perfect' shade of lipstick? Well now, you don't even have to set foot inside a shop, or embark on expensive trial-and-error. Many brands, from M.A.C. Cosmetics to Maybelline, Bobbi Brown to E.L.F. have launched a number of 'virtual try-on' opportunities, both online and in stores. Using incredibly clever technology, they layer shades onto your face using a 'FaceTime'-type technology.

These are great for seeing how a shade will flatter your complexion (or not). It can be fun to use one and work through a brand's entire shade portfolio for one product, to see just how everything from a pale beige lip to a deep purple look on you. You might be surprised!

The rules for what 'suits' you are all broken. Shade choice used to be based on eye colour/skin tone or whether you suited warm/cool shades, but that's only really relevant if you always wear the same foundation or skin base. Here are some tips, to help you choose:

- Have your normal 'face' on and your hair done, to get a proper picture of the effect of a new shade.

- You need a few 'grab and run' shades – colours that you buy time and again and that work on good and bad days. But don't get stuck in a rut. When you have more time for your make-up, enjoy experimenting. Build confidence by dabbing a new shade on top of your 'safe' shade to begin with. Take inspiration from seasonal trends. Especially if you have great, full lips, anything goes, and you can even wear the crazy, fab, of-the-moment daring colours and textures, as statements.

- It is always best to try lipstick on the lips, for a true idea of the colour. In a store, where tester products may be available, always ask for a disposable applicator with which to sweep the colour onto lips. If you don't want to try on your lips, for any reason, the pads of your fingers are the next-best place – they are a deeper shade that's not far off lip colour and they can be held up to your face. Of course, if you're TV shopping you can order to try in the comfort of your own home – even better!

- Stand back and look in a full-length mirror, or at least head and shoulders, and see how the lip colour looks from a distance. I'd like you to wear a colour that you can see and which complements your eye colour. Lip colour can make your eyes and complexion 'pop'.

- What are your favourite outfit colours? Are they warm tones: corals, browns, peaches, with gold jewellery? Or cool: pinks, blues, greys, with silver jewellery? All colour 'families' have a warm or a cool version, so it's definitely the easiest rule to follow: a red can be warm, with softer coral undertones, or cool, with bluish undertones. In general you will be one or the other, although a small percentage of people can get away with either/ both (when it comes to lipstick AND blusher). Warm/cool can be a good starting point, but at the same time, because so many of us mix things up on a daily basis now, with clothes and jewellery, rules can still be broken.

- Do also work to find your perfect nude – not insipid or bland, but colourful and engaging. This can be your 'younger-looking' lip shade, your most versatile colour that you will repeat buy for years and works with everything from a no-make-up look through to balancing the strength of a smoky eye. The heritage make-up artistry brands are reliably good at these shades, the most famous, of course, being Bobbi Brown.

LIPSTICK – NOT JUST FOR LIPS

If you have a great lip colour, a quick cheat is to touch it onto your fingertips and add a touch to eyes, in the socket line, blending well by patting it in. You can also dab a little on your cheekbones. This is fab for a quick make-up or casual/natural look, but also a great technique on top of other make-up if your sugar level dips and you start to look a bit wan mid-afternoon!

Paler skins can do this with an apricot, terracotta or peach shade, but reds, purple, strong pinks and burgundies work brilliantly on darker skin tones, for a fabulous 'pop' of colour.

Alison's Tip ————————————————

When you change your hair colour, you need to re-evaluate your lipstick choices, and indeed, your whole make-up. This should happen at menopause, too, when your hair and skin tone changes, often becoming paler. Don't keep wearing the same shade you did five or ten years ago – see it as an opportunity to experiment. Give yourself some time to adjust to your style, to help redefine your confidence. (See also Menopause, p.102.)

To lip-line... or not to lip-line?

One good reason to line your lips is to avoid lipstick running into the feathery lines that appear on our upper lips when we age. (Smokers or ex-smokers are often affected prematurely.) The waxy texture of the lipliner acts as a barrier to prevent your lipstick bleeding. You can also use it as a lip base to help lipstick stay put for longer, drawn all over your lips as if you were using a colouring book.

My advice is always to choose a lipliner that is just a tiny bit darker than the colour of your natural lips, rather than matching the colour of your lipstick. This is the best shade to 'over-paint' your lip line, to rebalance or emphasise your shape, which is something I especially like to do when I have time; it makes lips look fuller. You can then go over this with any lip colour or gloss. It takes a little practice, so spend some time in front of the mirror and see what a difference it can make.

Alternatively, check out 'invisible' lipliners, which are see-through, but create a waxy barrier to prevent lipstick bleeding. When you discover your perfect lip liner, buy in multiples – you won't want to be without it!

If you are suffering from feathery lip lines and lipstick bleeding, use your regular anti-ageing eye cream on the area around your lips, because the skin is similar and it can work to diminish the lines, just as it does around the eyes.

Alison's Tip ——————— ——————— ———————

Make like a pro! Professional make-up artists create wardrobes of lip colours by melting or 'smooshing' lipsticks into empty lipstick palettes or stackable pots; we can all do the same, with empty lipstick palettes/pots from make-up artist brands. This gives you all your lip shades visible at a glance, so you can create custom colours by blending together. If you're down to the stub of a lipstick, you can use a hairdryer to melt it into a palette, or into a little pot to carry with you.

THREE LIP LOOKS

There are so many different lip effects to play around with, but here are three that I return to, time and again…

- **A casual soft lip**
Easy-peasy for daywear.
Pick up colour with your fingertips from the lipstick bullet and pat onto lips, for a stain. That's it – done!

- **A volumised lip look**
If you feel you have 'thin' lips, this can make them appear a little plumper.

1. Cover the lips with foundation, powder foundation or lip primer.

2. Line the lips, extending slightly outside the outer lip line, if you like. To instantly make lips appear fuller, fill in the cupid's bow, above the centre of the top lip, so the lip line appears to go straight across – instant 'trout pout'!

3. 'Fill in' the lips with the same pencil just as if you were using a crayon in a colouring-in book.

4. For the illusion of an even fuller look, use the 'shadow' shade in your contour/bronzing palette, or a bronzer, and apply a little bit under the lower lip, blending well.

5. Add gloss to the centre of the bottom lip and mash lips together.

- **The whole (lip) works**

This ombré look will give a velvety finish, ideal for an evening look or when you need to look super-groomed.

1. Start as for the volumised lip, up to and including Step 4.

2. Apply lipstick either from the bullet or with a brush. Place a tissue between lips and press down on it, to create a long-lasting stain.

3. Apply a second coat of lipstick and a lighter tone in the middle; mash lips together.

4. Highlight with gloss in the centre of the bottom lip, for extra shine.

The right brows can work like a mini-facelift.

It's all about the brow

Brows have become big business in recent years, with products offering us so many different looks. The right brows can even work like a mini-facelift.

Brows are your face's architecture; they give it shape and definition. Colouring and shaping your brows can be one of the most transformative elements of your make-up regime. Brows can lift your face, make it look more awake, counteract the look of dark circles, enhance your hair colour and add structure to your make-up and hairstyle. There have been many fab brow product innovations in recent years, so I'm going to look at which might work best for you. Personally, I have a whole 'wardrobe' of brows. It's fun to experiment with different brow looks to see how they can transform your face and balance different make-up looks. Let's look at shaping first.

SHAPING

You may have brows that grow strongly, in which case keeping them tamed, trimmed and groomed is your big challenge. Or you may have fine, sparse, pale brows, which need emphasising. Here's what works best…

- **There are two types of brow hair.**
  There are the 'terminal' hairs, which form the brow itself and are pigmented. Then there are the 'vellous', feathery, generally almost invisible-to-the-eye hairs which grow on the skin underneath and around the terminal hairs.

- **At the very least, lightly tidy up your brows.**
  Even if you don't want to emphasise your brows for an anti-ageing effect or as a fashion statement, everyone benefits from simple

maintenance, using tweezers or brow removal wax. This means taking out any stray hairs growing between the two brows, above the nose (the 'monobrow' area); that applies to guys as well as women. You should also remove any of the little fuzzy or fine 'vellous' hairs growing beneath the natural brow, which sharpens the brow-line and has the effect of opening up the eyes. It will also give a smoother finish to your eye make-up. You can use tweezers, wax strips or little gizmos that are like mini-sanders for this (men love these, in my experience), but one caveat: never remove hairs from above the brow.

- **Consult a professional, for a brow 'blueprint'.**
Beauty salons, brow bars and beauticians can all professionally shape (and if required, tint) your brows; many barbers now offer brow-grooming services for men.

The key is to communicate the style of brow you want, just as you'd discuss a haircut with a hairdresser before they got out the scissors. Do also be clear how much time you have for brow make-up daily, so that the effort required matches your lifestyle. Brow technicians are highly competent, but if you want a natural shape rather than a structured, 'fashion' brow, SAY SO. Once you've had your brows professionally shaped, it's easier to do the upkeep at home.

Brow bars do a great job of maintenance but it requires a monthly appointment. Think about how that fits into your life, your budget and your look. (If you wear your hair off your face, brows are generally a higher priority than when you have a fringe.)

- **Use cellophane templates.**
These kits contain stencils which you place over the brows as a guideline, showing you where to pluck/shade to achieve the desired shape. They can be good for having a play around, but they don't work for everyone because your brows may just not fit the template.

- **How to tweeze.**

Make sure you're positioned in good light, with a good, non-magnifying mirror. (With a magnifying mirror you can overdo things.) With slant tweezers, pluck one or two hairs off one eye, then switch to the other and mirror the action on the other side, otherwise it's too easy to overdo one brow and then try to even up – you'll never manage it. If you have poor eyesight, it can be best to get your brows professionally shaped first, then when hairs grow back you can use a magnifying mirror to spot them.

- **How to wax.**

Use Vaseline or a skin balm on any hair you don't want to remove (the wax can't grab the Vaselined hairs). Then use a thin tool like an orange stick or a thin spatula saved from a skincare product for applying the wax to brow hairs with precision; the spatula provided with a waxing kit itself is usually way too big. Cut down any fabric strips for removing the wax, to around a centimetre wide, to avoid mistakes. Wax in stages; take off some hairs from both eyes, then assess things and decide if you want to take off more. 'Stretch' and support the skin with your other hand, while you're removing the hairs (this helps prevent bruising). Pull off the strips in the opposite direction of the hair growth.

Alison's Tip

Don't shape brows straight after a facial and avoid waxing or plucking when you're feeling hot, or your skin is feeling sensitive because it will hurt more. Don't embark on brow removal just before your period, because the pain factor's way higher.

SLANTY OR POINTY?

There are two types of tweezer: slant-ended and pointed. 'Beginners' should definitely start with the slant-ended, which have an edge about a quarter of a centimetre wide. Pointed tweezers are more precise and harder to master, but they are crucial if you have dark hair or stronger hair growth, in which case brows can look stubbly or like blackheads when they grow in, and you want to be able to grab them fast.

Invest in good tweezers (not the ones in a Christmas cracker). Ideally keep them in the tube they come in, or they'll get misshapen and will stop grabbing the hairs. Never, ever leave them loose in your make-up bag.

BROW SHADING

Brows aren't born equal. Your goal is to even them up to create facial symmetry. There's an absolute arsenal of products to help achieve this, available in a wide range of shades. Here are my tips, in order of easiness...

Brow gel

If you're nervous or just starting to shade your brows, this is the simplest of all. You can buy it in clear, to tame your natural brow, or tinted to add a touch of colour.

Brow mascara

Brilliant grab-and-run products, with a mascara-style wand and sometimes fibres to bulk up your natural brow density. Most ranges have a universal taupe shade, if you're unsure about which colour to go for. You can also find greys and auburn shades to match those hair colours. Great for guys to cover grey or counteract a tired look.

Pencils

These are good if you want to slightly alter the shape of your brow, as they are drawn directly onto skin beneath the brow hairs. A very wide shade range is available, but again, most brands have a 'universal' taupe which works on almost everyone. Always use short, feathery, light strokes and build the effect. You can also get super-fine pencils for very realistic, individual, feathery strokes. Go for propelling pencils or keep yours sharpened, to avoid scratching.

Brow pens

These come in two formats: a fine-tipped brush (akin to a liquid eyeliner brush), or a small, comb-like tip. They are designed to mimic the effect of microblading, a tattoo-like treatment that can create a brow that lasts for up to two years. (Microblading sounds like the answer to brow prayers – and if you've lost your brows, it really can be – but if you don't like the results, you're really stuck with them.) Stroked onto the brow area, they deliver feathery strokes, but they're not that easy to master and I'd advise starting with a lighter shade than normal, while you get the hang of the pen.

Brow shadows/powders

Powders generally come with a small, angled brush for applying directly to the brow hairs; nowadays they are very long-wearing and will stay put well. After you've applied the powder, run through the brow with a spoolie brush (a tool like a mascara brush), for a natural finish.

Brow pomade

A waxy product, again applied with an angled brush. These are my personal favourite. It sets so it's sweat-proof, hat-proof, waterproof so you don't need to retouch later in the day. You can also get your brows (and lashes) professionally 'laminated' to encourage the hairs to point in the right direction.

Alison's Tip

A polished, finished make-up look needs a stronger brow, and a light/natural make-up a lighter brow. If you do a strong brow when you're just wearing a dab of tinted moisturiser, you'll look like you've got a couple of slugs on your forehead and that's all anyone will see when they look at you.

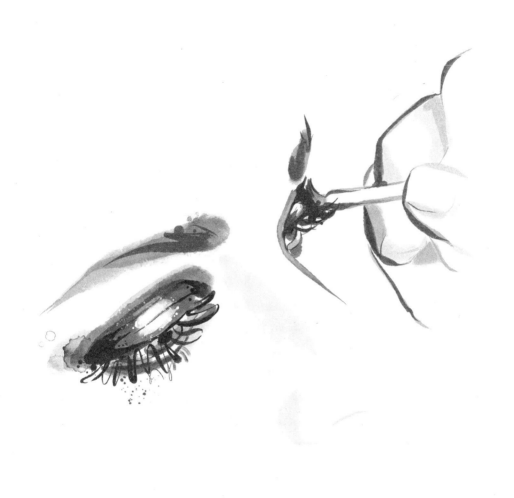

YOUR BROW WARDROBE

Before you start, remove any foundation that's been applied to the brow hairs when you did your base, using a cotton bud.

Brow One: The grab-and-run brow

This is the brow look for working from home, answering the door, going to the Post Office. It covers greys and fills in missing bits, without changing the shape of the brow.

1   Use a mascara wand-style brow product or a brow powder. You don't want to change the shape; simply work the product through the brow, first sweeping against the direction of hair growth (so it 'ruffles' the hairs). Concentrate in the middle and at the highest points.

2   Then apply again, working in the direction of hair growth to smooth down.

Brow Two: The meeting friends/going out/ job interview brow

To counteract tiredness and give an instant lift. This physically (but subtly) increases the size of the brow and lifts the eye.

1   Use a pencil. Draw short strokes onto the brows and skin to emphasise your brows, taking them a millimetre higher, following the natural curve.

2   Use pencil strokes to extend the end of the brow, following the natural line. (If you're older, you can take the line slightly upwards at the temple to lift.)

3   Sweep through with a spoolie brush, if you like, to soften the effect slightly.

Alison's Tip

You can get really good at-home kits for tinting, but (as with salon tinting appointments), you need a patch test 24 hours before use, to make sure you don't react. If it's the first time you've used a particular product, err on the side of caution and leave it on for a short time before removing the dye – it's easier to add colour than take it away. Always time your dye session; it's too easy to lose track. When time's up, wipe it off and assess the results; you can always reapply. Bear in mind that the dampness can make the brow look a little darker. If it's night-time, maybe wait till next day to get a proper look and you can revisit then.

Brow Three: The metropolitan brow

For a more groomed look, for special events. The aim is to create a shape that is wider, higher and longer than your natural brow. If you want to wear a smoky eye, you'll need this stronger brow look, for sure.

1   Use a brow pomade with an angled brow brush, or a fine brow pencil. Whichever product you choose, thicken the appearance of the brow with lots of angled upwards strokes of the brush, rather than going sideways along the grain of the brow.

2   Create a pointed shape at the arch (before the brow tapers downwards again). I create a definite outward angle here, slightly higher than the natural line, rather than following the natural downward curve.

3   Blend the product through with a spoolie brush and apply gel to set.

4   To accent the brow shape, apply highlighter below and above the brow with an eyeshadow brush, right up to the line of the brow itself.

Brow Four: The all-singing, all-dancing, going-out brow

Also known as the 'Instagram brow' because of its popularity among influencers. It's fully angled and lengthened, more groomed-looking and stronger to match a more structured, glamorous look, and is best done before foundation on the rest of your face, as it's the main focus.

1   First, use a cotton bud to clean the brow.

2   Use a spoolie brush to groom, brushing with upward strokes.

3   As for the metropolitan brow, use a fine brow pencil or pomade with angled brow brush to thicken the appearance of the brow with lots of angled upward strokes.

4   Take the product along the brow, creating a pointed shape at the arch and angle slightly higher than the natural line.

5   Blend through with a spoolie brush and apply gel to set.

6   Using a concealer brush, apply foundation around the brow to frame it. Press into the skin with fingertips or a blender.

7   Apply highlighter above and below the brow with an eyeshadow brush to accent the shape.

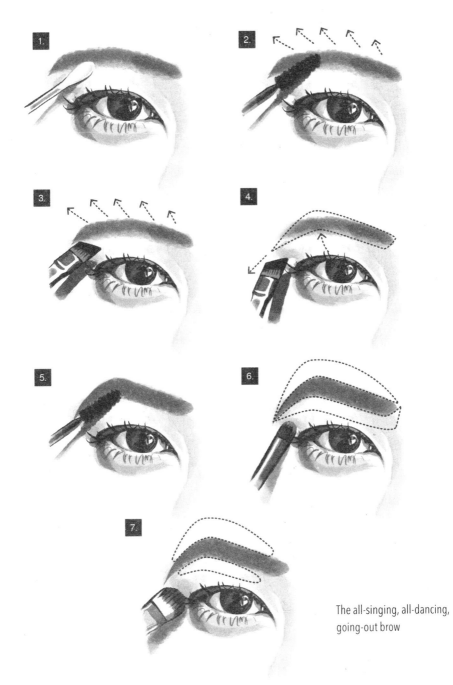

The all-singing, all-dancing, going-out brow

Bright eyes

When someone looks at you, they notice your eyes first. The right make-up showcases your eyes, upping their sparkle factor...

In this section, I'm going to look at the vast array of eye make-up products out there, from bases and primers, to sticks, pens and shadows.

Start with a base

Eye bases work to even out lid discolouration and counteract the look of tiredness, and can be very useful if your eye make-up creases or disappears; if you like vibrant, fashion colours, you'll definitely want to use one of these. Your first port of call is to use your regular medium-to-full coverage concealer – concealer is better than foundation here as it's more opaque. Smooth into lids with a beauty blender. A good eye base has a bit of 'grip'; be aware that if your regular concealer is too moisturising, it will slide off, in which case try an eye primer. You can also get lifting and firming eye primers, for the more mature eye, and all-in-one eye primers that incorporate colour.

Eye pencil or shadow stick

Chunky pencils, cream eye sticks and kajals/kohl pencils can create a natural effect and are a cinch to use. Draw onto your skin and blend with a finger or a sponge-tipped eye tool; you've got 30 seconds of smudge-time, at least, before it sets. For a daily look, this may be all you need. They're also great in hot weather. Dark shades can be used as a liner, or blend out with a synthetic brush/smudger tip for a smoky eye look. Kajals/kohls can also be used on the eye waterline.

Cream shadow

Also very versatile, these come in tubes, some with doe-foot applicators, or small pots (use a sponge applicator or fingers with the latter). Good for highlighting the brow bone (see p.202). For a really simple look, just smooth onto lids in a neutral taupey shade, add mascara, and job done. You can now find cream shadows with tightening/firming lid benefits, too.

Powder shadows

You always need brushes for these. A small, stubby domed brush is best for applying an intense layer of shadow near the lashes, and a soft, fluffy blender brush for shaping and shading. You can use some powder shadows dry or wet. Used wet, they can work as an eyeliner. Used dry, they are good to 'set' a gel liner. Play with different techniques when you're in a Make-up Toybox mood.

Tone on tone

For most people, nudes and browns are the most flattering, go-to shades. The right nudes will brighten the eyes, so if your nudes make you look tired, sorry, but you need to throw that palette away! There are some absolutely fantastic nude palettes out there (and very affordable, too), which offer huge versatility for all skin tones (try artistry brands that offer hundreds of nudes).

If you want to wear fashion shades, nude can still be your eyeshadow 'underwear', perhaps with your bolder shade blended around the lashes. You *can* wear primary colours, a flash of orange or green, or pink or blue eyeliner, whatever your skin tone or age. A fun way to try a fashion look, without scaring yourself, is to add a flash of coloured eyeliner: apply your usual dark liner at lash level, then a flash of coloured liner above that. Take time at your Make-up Toybox to play around.

If you feel stuck in a rut with your neutrals, this is where you might want to make a bee-line for a consultant at a make-up counter who looks different to you. The experts can teach you something finger-on-the-pulse, make-up fashion-wise, sharing tips and techniques to update your look. Try applying fashion colours in the middle of the eyelid, blended over your 'safe' nude. Remember: it's make-up, not a tattoo; it comes off again, so there is no risk! Enjoy it.

Eye-sculpting how-to

If you have a double lid (as I do), where your upper lid is hooded and droops to the eyelash line, these techniques will help disguise that and create the illusion of a socket line. You can also use the bronzer technique, which is a little quicker, for a casual daytime look.

The bronzer technique

Stand back from the mirror, look straight ahead, and with a long-handled, fluffy eyeshadow brush, create a socket using a matte bronzer suited to your skin tone. Irrespective of where your natural socket is, you literally fake one, mid-way between brow and lash-line. Sweep the brush back and forth, making sure the results are seamlessly blended.

The eyeshadow technique

1 Within your eyeshadow palettes, find a flesh or skin tone that's a bit darker than your complexion. Using an eyeshadow blender brush, staring straight ahead, build a socket line on the outer third of the eye towards the brow, to counterbalance the drooping of the eye. This widens and lifts the eye.

2 Brush on a paler shade of shadow underneath and above this 'fake' socket.

3 Then brush the darker colour inwards, to soften – and you've got a new socket line. Balance with a darker eyeliner too, if you wish.

4 With a clean brush, buff the light colour outwards, above and below the darker colour, for a smooth finish.

Alison's Tip

Use eyeshadow brushes, not the brushes that come with your shadows – they're too small, fiddly and they don't give the seamless effect that dedicated shadow brushes do. The longer handled ones are easier for creating a pro finish.

Bronzer technique

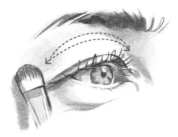

Eyeshadow technique

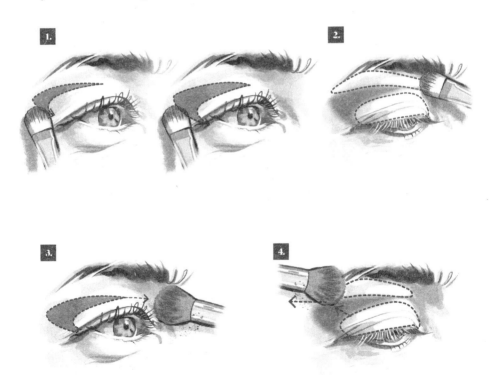

Eye-sculpting how-to: two techniques for hooded eyelids

EYELINER MASTERCLASS

Eyeliner is amazing for giving definition to eyes, creating the illusion of greater lash length and making eyes appear larger. These are the four key techniques and the products you'll need, ranging from a casual, quick look to a cat-flick or a smoky eye for a more 'dressed-up' effect.

Look 1: Natural/day make-up

Take an eyeliner pencil or a kajal/kohl pencil and apply it along the upper waterline (between your lashes and the eye itself), for a 'lifted' look.

Look 2: Casual smoky eye

A super-easy, quick way to create a smoky eye is using a kajal pencil, not only on the inner waterline but on the lid, smudged outwards using a small blender brush or fingers. Alternatively, some of these kajal pencils have a built-in sponge smudger tip, in which case, use that.

Look 3: Building a smoky eye

1. This builds on Look 2. Use a fine-tipped shadow brush to layer a deep eyeshadow over the pencil for extra depth, blending as you go. Make sure the shading on the upper and lower lids joins at the outer corner; some of us have a crease line here which needs to be deliberately filled in.

2. Blend the shadow and liner upwards towards the socket line, building a wider, higher eye.

Look 4: Liquid liner/cat flick

1. Applying one sweep of liquid liner is tricky if you don't have a steady hand. Instead, press the length of the brush onto the lashes at intervals, joining up the dashes as you go.

2. You can extend this with an angled cat-flick line at the corner – always upwards, on a mature face, to 'lift' your eyes.

3. You can then 'fill in' the cat-flick at the outer corner, to make it thicker, if you like that look. Look downwards for a few seconds to allow the liquid eyeliner to dry without smudging. You can also set the look by applying a matching powder over the top.

Natural make-up

Casual smoky eye

Cat flick

Building a smoky eye

Eyeliner masterclass: four key techniques

MASCARA IS YOUR BEST FRIEND...

Finding your perfect mascara match is almost always a matter of trial and error, till you find out the wand and formula that works for you. And I'm afraid you'll spend a fair bit of money along the way, because there's no 'magic wand' solution here – literally!

There are as many as seven different 'lash types', well-understood by make-up brands, but never communicated to customers. What that results in is a huge, baffling spectrum of mascara brushes, including fibre, rubber, and those created by 3-D printing. Add to that different formulas to curl, lengthen, separate, volumise and you've countless permutations. Even mascaras that promise to work on everyone just don't; a product that grips your lashes might simply skate off someone else's. The bottom line is that there are thousands of different permutations of pigment and brush and formula, which is why it's so challenging to find your perfect match. Add to that the fact that for some people, some mascaras make their eyes water or trigger sensitivity, something you won't know until you've tried a product out. If you have very sensitive eyes, look for ranges which make the claim to be 'hypoallergenic', although even then, sensitivity CAN happen. You can also try vegan or 'free from' formulas.

Once you've found a mascara that works for you, if you want a change (or that product is discontinued, which is so frustrating), look for a near-identical wand, next time. A perfect mascara match is about wand first, formulation second. Here are my top tips:

- **It's all about black mascara, nowadays.**
  Mascara colours come and go but black really is the 'Little Black Dress' of mascara. It goes with everything. If you do like brown mascara, check the shade doesn't have too much red in it, which will make eyes look tired.

- **Size matters.**
  If you've got small eyes and skinny lashes, buy skinny brushes. If you've got lots of lashes and big eyes, big, fat brushes will almost

certainly work better for you. If you use a big brush on a small eye, you'll spend more time clearing up the mess with a cotton bud later.

- **Bobble-tipped wands can be brilliant for accessing inner and outer lashes.**
Most people miss those but enhancing those extra 5mm on the inner corners of your lashes works instantly to make eyes look bigger. The same applies on the outer lashes, which are often missed.

- **Lash curlers are love-it-or-hate-it tools.**
I find them torture. If you do want to use one, invest in a premium brand, and use carefully (always before mascara), otherwise they can tug out clumps of lashes. If your lashes naturally droop or are straight, do try curlers, or look for specific curling mascaras. You can also get them professionally permed.

- **Waterproof mascaras are on the way out.**
The days of a separate formula which you used for emotional or rainy days or for swimming are behind us; instead, look for 'long-wear' or 'water-resistant'. Those old waterproof formulas were a nightmare to remove and damaged lashes, so they broke off. You might also look for 'tube' mascaras, which coat the lashes with little tubes of product and come off with warm-to-hot water rather than remover. They stay put really well.

- **Use your freshest mascara on upper lashes.**
If you have an older mascara, use it on lower lashes where you're more likely to get clumping with a fresh mascara. Lower lashes need less coverage.

- **Grab the lashes by the root and sweep through to tips.**
Wiggle the brush at the root. Then move your head slightly to the side to do the next section of lashes, wiggling and then sweeping root to tip. Turn your head to get to your lashes, rather than fiddle around with the position of the wand while keeping your head still.

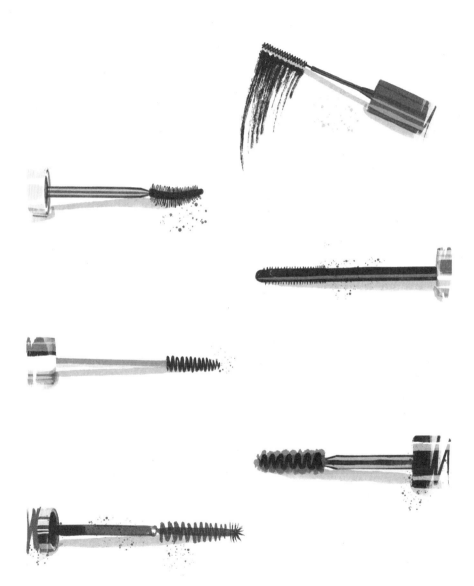

• **Use powder or powder foundation to make your mascara stay in place longer.**

Most daily mascaras are long-lasting, but if yours smudges easily, take a big powder brush or a fluffy eyeshadow brush, dip it in face powder, tap it sharply to remove excess, and sweep it over your lashes before applying mascara. Some people have oilier eyelids which leads to smudging; if that's you, avoid oily skincare on your eyes, even the night before. If you try the tricks above and still get smudges, try having your lashes tinted instead. You won't get the glamorous volume, but these are great on pale, grey or red lashes.

• **Tints, perms and inserts.**

For a longer-lasting solution, you can get eyelashes tinted, permed or get inserts (available in beauty salons and via beauty therapists), which requires upkeep every six weeks or so. Perming 'lifts' droopy lashes; inserts actually boost the volume of lashes.

THE MASCARA EYE LIFT

By 'lifting' your lashes, this technique can make eyes look wider, brighter – and younger. Great for tired days or mature eyes.

1. Start with a skinny brush mascara, whatever your lash type, wiggling it from root to tip in zig-zag motions, making sure to coat the base of the lashes to help create the illusion of thickness at the root.

2. Then concentrate on the outer area (switch to a mascara with a thick wand if you have thicker lashes), using the brush to lift the lashes at the outer half of the eye.

3. By now, there'll be less product on the wand, which makes it perfect for doing your lower lashes.

4. Don't overlook the fine lashes, top and bottom, right at the inner and outer corner of the eye.

Alison's Tip

If you have your hair tied back from your face while you're doing your make-up, it will probably look quite strong. If so, shake your hair out the way it's going to look, and see what needs balancing – your make-up will almost certainly look much less strong, but you can balance it out based on what hairstyle, outfit and neckline you'll be wearing.

Ask Alison: make-up Q&A

You asked. (Or your best friend did.) So here are the answers…

Q: Why can't I get the full foundation coverage I've seen on social media?

This is either down to a) the skincare you use underneath or b) your application technique. If you layer on a lot of products in the morning – serum, foundation/SPF – then let that sink in for 20–30 minutes before applying foundation, because it won't 'grab' onto the skin otherwise. If you're using fingers for application, that can be the reason: fingertip application gives you light-to-medium coverage at best, so switch to a foundation brush/stipple brush for a fuller finish.

Q: How can I tell the level of coverage offered by a concealer?

To gauge the opacity, apply it to any blue veins or age spots on the back of your hand. Some concealers can literally make them vanish before your eyes; others are more sheer. Then you can make up your mind.

Q: Does make-up cause spots?

It can, if you put it on the wrong way. First of all, always wash your hands before you do your make-up. Foundations should be applied *downwards* so they glide over pores and don't push product into it. Applicators should be washed regularly so that you have a clean one daily, to avoid contamination. Look for make-up products that are clay-based, with 'clean' or 'free from' formulas and (particularly in the case of foundations and concealers) may have anti-blemish ingredients. Always take your make-up off when you get home.

Q: Lipstick colours never come up true on me...

This is usually down to your individual pH levels; some people just change everything to bright pink! It really can happen. You can try putting foundation over your lips as a buffering layer before lip colour, or buy a specific lip primer. Or try shopping with one of the 'artistry' make-up brands, as these are designed to stay true.

Q: What can I do about eyeshadow that creases?

This can be the result of a naturally oily eyelid, or related to crêpiness. Try using concealer on your lid, invest in an eye primer, or try one of the all-in-one liquid primer shadows, if you don't mind switching from your regular eyeshadow palette. You can also try a shadow with a clay in it, to absorb the oil. If you use rich, moisturising eye products, this can also be a cause: switch from a cream to a gel in the mornings.

Q: My mascara/eyeliner run and smudge...

This can be caused by an oily eye make-up remover or cleanser the night before, or a too-rich eye cream. Switch to a gel eye treatment for the mornings; you can double-dose on your rich night cream the night before if you're worried the eye zone isn't getting enough nourishment. If that doesn't work, use a touch of loose powder or oil-absorbing powder before applying mascara; apply with a small brush, tapping it first to remove any excess, and run it over the lid and lashes. Your mascara and eyeliner will then 'take' better without any oily residue underneath.

Q: How do I make my make-up last longer for a wedding/ photograph/special occasion/job interview/whatever...

Load up your skincare the night before, especially with serums or hydrating masks, so that your skin is plumped and hydrated. On the morning of the big event, you want just a light moisturiser, so that you can concentrate on priming the skin and layering on make-up. At every stage of the make-up, 'set' creamy textures with a powdery product, for make-up that is long-wear and sweat-proof. Oily, creamy textures make everything slide off the face, so set foundation and blusher with powders. Layer a gel/liquid eyeliner with a matching eyeshadow powder. For the lips, use a lip primer, then draw all over the lips with a lip-toned lip pencil and blot that by biting onto a tissue to mattify further, before adding lip colour. If you find your make-up is 'sitting' on the surface too much, press into the skin with warm hands.

Q: I'm allergic to all mascaras – help!

Have you tried free-from or vegan brands? Many of them have gentle ingredients, with shorter ingredients lists. Always do a patch test (see p.253), though that won't really tell you whether your eyes will react or not. As an alternative, try salon lash tinting or professional lash inserts. If that's too much of an expense or faff, create the optical illusion of thicker eyelashes and a more defined eye with eye liner.

Q: If I have a lip or eye infection, do I need to get rid of my make-up?

First off, if you have a cold sore or a stye on your eye you should avoid wearing make-up on those areas. Powder textures aren't a problem because they are dry, and bacteria need moisture to breed. If you must apply make-up to the infected area, use a clean cotton bud for application and throw it away afterwards. If you're using an eye pencil, sharpen it between doing one eye and the next (and immediately after the infected eye). When I've suffered from eye infections, I've used disposable applicators which are easy to buy on the internet.

Q: Do I need a make-up setting spray?

For me, the jury's out. If you follow the long-lasting make-up tips above, and you're not wearing anything over your face, you shouldn't need one. In my experience, some setting sprays have too high a water content, which in turn (ironically) makes your make-up dehydrate more quickly. The newer formulas are better, and with the advent of regular mask-wearing they may be worth a try.

Q: I have poor eyesight and it's tricky to apply make-up...

Oh, me too (I have to put my lenses in when I've finished my make-up). I had a very moving experience with a visually impaired client who came to London for the first time on her own with her guide dog, to get some make-up advice from me, so I know how important this is to many people.

My first suggestion (if you do have some sight) would be to get hold of a good magnifying glass – as strong as you need. Go for looks which are less complex, e.g. a pencil eyeliner you can blur rather than a cat-flick liquid liner. Choose cream-to-powder textures which are easier and more foolproof than powders and keep to single shades; smooth them onto the contours of the eye, feeling your way around. A gel or cream blusher also lets you feel exactly where you're applying it.

The consultants on make-up counters in department stores and beauty boutiques just love to advise in situations like this – or a private room in a beauty salon, if you prefer – and are perfectly poised to give advice on the types of shades and textures that will flatter and be easy for you to work with. I promise you: they'll bend over backwards to help.

Hair

"

Every day can be a Great Hair Day

Crowning glory or daily nightmare? With huge technological advances in products and accessories, every day really can be a Great Hair Day, I promise!

My very first job made me incredibly aware of how central hair is to people's self-esteem. As a beauty therapist and make-up artist working within a hair salon, I used to sweep the floors and make coffees, chatting to customers to tempt them to visit my treatment room. I'd see people walking in with their shoulders down, and after a great hairstyling session, stand taller and walk out ready to look the world right in the eye again.

Aside from the usual hair challenges many of us experience, about 20 years ago I lost a lot of my hair through a thyroid condition. I was on TV and hosting beauty events, busy, busy, and I noticed that it had gone very thin and ratty. I couldn't put it up in a ponytail and colour didn't work properly. It took around 10 years to get back to where it had been, as my health improved and I found supplements and minerals that boosted my hair health.

For many years it was all about disguising that hair loss, for me; at one point, I'd lost about an inch all around my hairline and so I learned all about volumising tricks, techniques and products. Trust me: those were nowhere near as good as they are now. Mousses, back then, were sticky and itchy, unlike today's, which leave your hair soft, shiny, bouncy and oomphy.

My hairdresser was so, so helpful at that difficult time in my life. I don't think I realised how it had dented my confidence until things were back to normal, all those years later. We go to hair salons not just for haircuts and blow-dries but for relaxation and therapy. Because hair *is* so bound up with confidence, your hairdresser really is a Very Important Person in your life. Treasure them. Buy them a Christmas present and a no-reason-at-all present if you find something you think they'll like. If you know they like their coffee from a particular coffee bar, pick one up for them on your way to an appointment. Tip them generously. A good hairdresser is worth their weight in gold. Although this isn't true for everyone, they can also be your emotional dumping ground, almost like a counsellor you tell your secrets to – maybe more than you'll tell your best friend.

You don't need to go to a fancy 'designer' hair salon to get a great haircut and colour, though. In fact, I've had some of the worst haircuts in my life at expensive London salons. Always ask around for salon recommendations. If you see someone whose style or hair colour you like, I promise they'll be flattered if you stop and ask them where they get their hair done. There are some truly fantastically talented people working as home hairdressers, a flexible lifestyle choice that lets them drop their kids off on the school run or work around holidays.

Many salons will have someone on the team who's best at dealing with coils and curls; always ask to see that person, or you might live where you can go to a specialist salon.

Communicate, communicate, communicate is the hairstyling mantra. Pump your stylist and colourist for wisdom and insights into your hair and what's best for you personally. I can't possibly advise you on the best style for you, or the products to help you achieve that at home – but they can.

Make sure your stylist/colourist understands your lifestyle and the amount of time you can set aside for daily hair maintenance – it's as important to get a cut and style that slots into your life, as it is to get one that suits your face shape. Your hairdresser can also share advice on how to prevent your styling regime from causing damage – if that straight style needs hot irons to sleek it to smoothness, what products do they recommend to counterbalance the drying effect of the heat, and its possible impact on your colour?

Don't get stuck in a rut, though – our hairstyle often needs to change if weight goes up and down, or we have a new job that means we're wearing different clothes. It's fun and exciting to have a change, from time to time.

And the great thing with hair, nowadays, is that anything goes. You don't have to go for a weekly shampoo and set, as our mothers did, or hide your grey. You can shave it all off. Dye it pink. Or ignore it completely and pin it up with a knitting needle, if you really can't be bothered.

And isn't that just brilliant?

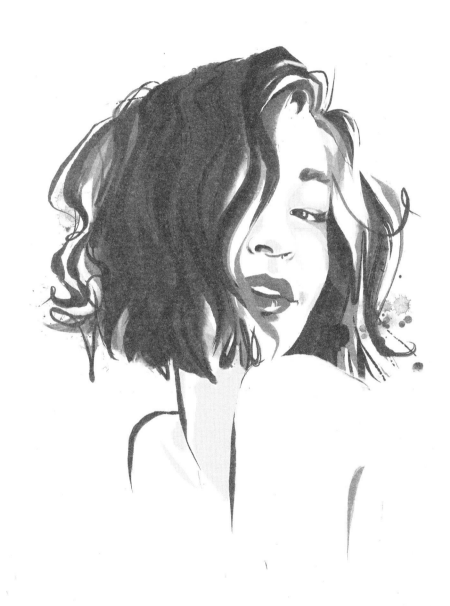

The ages and stages of hair

Just like skin, our hair and scalp evolve over the years. Here's how to keep shining on…

Like everything else that happens to our bodies, hair changes as we age. Hair, of course, has its roots (literally) in the scalp, which is affected by hormones, just like the skin on our faces. Teenage over-production of oil may slow down, but then other challenges arrive: the hormonal rollercoaster of pregnancy or menopause also take their toll. Stress has an impact, too. And while some changes are inevitable, some are the result of what we put our hair through on a regular basis: colouring, curling, straightening, taut ponytails…

As we age, hair follicles and the hair shaft start to shrink, which can lead to thinner hair and hair loss. (The rate of this loss, like male pattern baldness, can be hereditary.) You may notice yours isn't growing as fast or as thick as it once did. The stages I talk about here are a guide, but some people experience signs of ageing hair early. Whatever stage you're at, though, there's a lot you can do to support your hair, and even make it look and behave younger.

THE TEEN YEARS

Teenage hair is often oilier hair. Strictly, though, it's the scalp that's oily; this is an echo of what may be happening on your face, with over-productive sebum glands as a result of hormonal activity. You might not think so, but it's actually a good thing: those oils are like natural moisturisers and shine serums, so whether or not oiliness is a problem really depends on how fine or thick your hair is. If it's thick, use a bristle-style brush to disperse the oils through from root to tip; the natural oils will make your hair gleam. If it's fine, though, the greasiness can be very obvious, and the more you brush it, the more visible that will be.

If greasy hair makes you distressed — many people find that it makes them feel or look 'dirty' — then more frequent washing is the answer.

Check out clay-based shampoos and treatments, which draw oil from the scalp. Dry shampoo is your friend, and saves spending ages washing and styling. Spritz onto the root area, where the shampoo will absorb both oil and sweat, and this will help to take away the appearance of greasiness and make hair look thicker and more volumised, too.

In my experience, teens fall into two camps with their hair: the wash-and-go person, who leaves their hair to dry naturally, and the person who spends literally hours on their hair (and sometimes won't even leave their room, never mind the house, until it's the way they want it). Colour, cut, product, gunk: there's a lot of trial and (sometimes) error going on, and it may well be taking its toll, because the most destructive thing you can do is over-expose hair to heat, via tongs, curling irons and driers.

If you're really keen to experiment, why not put yourself in the hands of a hairdresser…? With their outsider's eye and insights into hair types and face shapes, they can steer you towards a style and/or colour that works for you and save a lot of that trial and error. (Unless you love the trial and the occasional error, of course.) It doesn't have to cost a fortune; most hairdressers offer training nights with their junior stylists/colourists, under the watchful gaze of their bosses. It's certainly less risky than trying things out for yourself at home. Colleges and hairdresser training schools also offer training evenings, so do some research, sign up, and make the most of these very affordable opportunities.

This is the time to get to grips with your hair texture. The oil levels may change, but if your hair is fine, it will stay fine. If it's coarser or thicker, that's how it will remain for a lifetime. The earlier you learn how to manage your own hair's particular quirks, the better.

TWENTY SOMETHING

Be grateful. Enjoy! Because the 100,000–150,000 strands that cover your scalp are probably the healthiest they'll ever be; hair growth really is optimal at this stage in life. If you do suffer from damage, it's probably the result of dabbling with hair colour changes and/or using too much heat on your hair. You've probably had plenty of style mistakes, colour disasters, had your hair cut short and hated it... We've all been there.

The key is to keep hair healthy, which depends on you getting a full range of vitamins and minerals in your diet. Among the essentials for shiny, strong hair are biotin (a B vitamin), zinc, iron, vitamins A, C, E, folic acid and protein: hair is actually made of a protein called keratin, and if you don't get enough in your diet, it can impact on your hair (and nails). If you're veggie or vegan, there are plenty of non-meat/non-fish sources of protein, such as tofu, lentils, beans, soya milk, nuts and nut butters etc.

You can be quite time-poor in your 20s, juggling the demands of jobs, a social life, perhaps settling down and starting a family (see the next section, too). In which case, cut yourself some slack: get organised on the haircare front to make life that little bit easier for yourself. Get into a routine: bulk-buy products that work for you, and line up your haircare near the shower so you don't waste a second looking for things. If you're working out at the gym, slap on a hair mask and shower it out afterwards. Ditto, if you're swimming; the heat under a swimming cap will help the mask to penetrate efficiently. If you're starting to earn a good salary, look at investing some of it in hair accessories that are perhaps kinder to hair: straightening irons with less damaging plates, hairdryers that dry more quickly (reducing exposure to heat), Velcro rollers which you can pin into hair and leave there while you do other things. (Confession time: I often drive to the TV studio wearing my Velcro rollers.)

Again, your hairdresser is your friend, who can point out any damage to your hair – maybe you've over-coloured it, or over-back-combed, maybe the grip you're using to pin your hair up is too sharp and is damaging the hair, or perhaps you're twiddling it anxiously while at the computer or commuting. It's easier to nip bad habits in the bud, if you learn about them early.

This isn't the time, yet, for heavyweight buttery masks and oils. A weekly mask with a cream-gel texture will work wonders, though, over and above shampoo and regular conditioner. NB Men benefit from using conditioner, too.

Alison's Tip

We now have countless 'eco' and sustainable haircare options, including styling products, which can perform just as well as 'traditional' products. Shampoo bars, which are like soap bars for the hair, are available for different hair types, and inexpensively priced. They're not for everyone, but if you're treading more lightly on the planet nowadays, why not see how you get on with them?

THIRTY SOMETHING

I'm going to talk about pregnancy here – the hormonal impact of pregnancy lasts for much longer than you'd think – a full two years, so don't expect your hair to get back to normal for quite some time. And if you're having IVF treatment, this is highly likely to affect your hair, too, which may become greasier, drier or thinner, or just behave differently.

During pregnancy itself, many women find that their hair becomes thicker. It's part of that famous 'blooming' look. This is because the normal hair fallout cycle slows down. Every (non-pregnant) day, we shed up to 100 hairs, but this slows almost to zero for someone who's expecting. Then, within a few months of the baby's appearance, the normal cycles resume and all those hairs you've been hanging onto are shed, even sometimes in quite significant clumps, which sends many women into a panic and impacts on self-confidence, even though it's a natural process.

Many women are concerned about colouring their hair in pregnancy. According to NHS guidance, it's perfectly safe – but of course, it's your call. If you do want to give up your colouring regime, talk to your hairdresser about how to manage the regrowth, if your colour's the permanent type – perhaps with a shorter/different style or a vegetable-based hair tint.

You may find that you want to switch to a more natural haircare range, in which case there are now many different options, including SLS- and SLES-free products. (Natural food stores are a great source for these.)

HAIR LOSS

If you're female and suffering from hair loss and it's not pregnancy-related, there can be other factors you might want to consult a doctor about. It can happen as a result of dieting, stopping hormone contraception, autoimmune disorders, polycystic ovary syndrome, iron deficiency or stress. For men, meanwhile, male pattern baldness is normal, but if you're losing hair fast, or suddenly, and it is not happening in the usual places (crown of the head, receding hairline), again, you might consult your GP to see if there's a medical reason for this.

Many parents are now switching to all-natural products as a lifestyle choice for their young families, too.

Above all, eat well. Make sure your vitamin intake is optimum (see above). After you've had the baby, you may want to supplement with specific formulas for skin, hair and nails. If you're really worried about ongoing hair loss, mention it to your doctor who can do a blood test to make sure you're not iron deficient and may be able to offer nutritional advice; if not, consider a nutritionist or trichologist. There are also topical drops for the scalp, featuring peptides, minerals and vitamins, that can be massaged into areas of hair weakness with the idea of stimulating faster regrowth.

Hair lost to pregnancy will almost certainly regrow, although one of the visible effects is an initial halo of baby-fine regrowth along the hairline; your hairdresser can advise on a style that will help deal with this, if it bothers you. Hair powders, which work like eyeshadows, are great to sweep into the thinner areas for an illusion of thickness.

FORTY SOMETHING

One challenge for this stage is related to dwindling hormone levels, as peri-menopause kicks in. This is the phase before menopause itself, often many years before your periods stop, when many people start to notice that hair is looking and feeling thinner, with the arrival of greys. Shrinking of the follicles begins, with the result that hair strands themselves may be thinner, and we have fewer of them. At any one time on our heads, we have follicles in resting, growing and shedding phases. As oestrogen levels dip, the number of follicles in the shedding and resting phases increases – hence the thinning. Again, make sure you're getting the right nutrients, particularly enough B-complex vitamins and biotin.

Once again, it's time to turn to your hairdresser. If you've always worn your hair straight, layers can create the illusion of fullness, especially in tandem with volumising products. Regular trims can keep the ends blunt, rather than wispy, and create an appearance of health and fullness. If you have dark hair and it's thinning, consider going lighter: there's less visible contrast between the hair and your scalp. A professional colourist can give you the truly personal advice that I can't, on this. You can also give the impression of thicker hair with scalp sprays, root lifting sprays and hair 'shadow powders' (literally they work like eyeshadows, but for the scalp). These are used after blow-drying to temporarily colour the scalp so that it's not so visible between thinned hair – an optical illusion, but it works.

FIFTY SOMETHING PLUS

By now, oestrogen levels are dropping off dramatically, and hair may continue to become thinner. And those oil glands – which were so super-active when we were teenagers – become lazier, which can lead to scalp tightness, itchiness and drier, courser, more brittle hair. Give yourself regular scalp massages with the pads of the fingers, to stimulate blood supply (which has the side benefit of helping to destress, too). If you're on medication (particularly for disease, or to lower lipids), hair loss may be a side-effect; a combination of medications may also result in loss, so do check with your pharmacist and speak to your doctor.

You're almost certain to be experiencing age-related pigment changes, too. Cells stop producing so much pigment, and eventually even the most resilient chestnut mane will become thinner, finer and greyer.

Well, the first big favour you can do your hair is to make sure you're eating healthily and keeping vitamin and mineral levels at optimum levels, perhaps through specific, targeted supplements. Healthy hair foods include spinach and other leafy green vegetables, eggs, fatty fish and antioxidant-rich berries, like strawberries, raspberries and blueberries.

The second big favour, quite simply, is to treat your hair with plenty of TLC. Gentle is better, at this stage in life. We tend to lose hair in particular through the action of washing, so perhaps reduce the number of times each week you do that. For more suds, just add extra water. Don't do things to hair that put it under undue stress – intense heat styling tools and too-tight ponytails being a case in point. Always apply a heat-protective product when styling, which provides a protective coating between your heated devices and the hair, and can help replenish moisture in the hair shaft. Avoid caustic chemicals like perms (your mother really was wrong about perming at 'a certain age'!), and over-exposure to harsh bleaches. The most rejuvenating addition to your haircare regime is a hair serum or a priming balm, to be applied to hair before you blow-dry. It can make your hair look and behave younger.

Yet again, your hairdresser is your go-to for advice on the least damaging, most flattering way to colour your hair. Alternatively, you may, as many more people are doing, choose to embrace the grey, which is now seen as a cool fashion statement. For much more about that, see p.232.

Alison's Tip

If it ain't broke, don't switch it! The time to trade up to more expensive products is if your regular shampoo and conditioner just aren't delivering results. If you're getting the right amount of gloss, shine and bounce from your products, there's no need to switch. But hair changes, as we age and at season changes, so haircare sometimes needs to change, too.

THE BALD TRUTH

Today, there are trichologists, specialist hair clinics, laser clinics and hair transplants to help to tackle male pattern baldness and female hair loss too. The technology behind products targeted at thinning hair has also advanced apace: there are thickening products that deliver lift and the illusion of volume, products with tiny fibres that temporarily boost hair's thickness, as well as scalp stimulating drops. All of these, though, cost money and/or time.

You can also choose to make your new hair pattern a style statement. Keep it short, with a No.1, a No.2 or even a fully shaved head – these are looks that have become hugely fashionable, not least through the world of football and music, where it's often a positive choice for a 'look' rather than a covering-up-the-bald-head choice. More women are proudly bearing fully shaved heads these days too. I know plenty of men who've shaved their heads for charity, loved the feeling and stuck with it. Short hair works with a close shave, or a full beard. Enjoy styling your beard/ stubble area, instead of your hair.

Finding your perfect haircare

We always seem to want the opposite of what we have! People with fabulous curls long for sleek, straight looks. Those with straight hair want to curl their hair into soft waves...

Well, the biggest single piece of advice I can give anyone about their hair is: the more you try to fight what nature gave you, the more time and money you'll need to devote to daily upkeep and maintenance. The good news? Whether you want to fight your hair's natural tendencies or go with the flow, shampoos, conditioners and styling products have never been better.

It really is all about ingredients. Since those days sweeping the floor in hair salons, I've seen huge leaps forward in haircare technology so that you really can make hair look and behave younger. At the same time, natural products have improved massively, so if you prefer botanical or 'free-from' options, there are no compromises to be made there, either. You can choose whether you want to buy from an organic haircare line, a trichologist's range or one created by one of the top-name hairstylists. The one piece of advice I'd give about the stylists' ranges though, is: do your homework and check out whether they use those products in their own salons. (You'll often get a clue from their social media accounts.) If not...? Enough said.

We all need a capsule hair 'wardrobe' – go-to products for day-to-day care – and it's really all dictated by your natural hair thickness and texture:

FINE HAIR

Fine hair refers to the thickness of the strand itself: skinny, fine and sometimes fragile, soft, and sometimes almost fluffy. You can have a lot of fine hair, so it appears thick, or more sparse hair. You may well have to wash your hair daily, in order for it not to go lank; in this case, you want to look for lightweight textures. A light shampoo will work best for you. Too-rich products can weigh hair down. Fine hair can be prone to splitting, but you may find a leave-in conditioner, spritzed onto the ends, helps. Many masks are almost certainly going to be too heavy for you, weighing the hair down. Instead, look for pre-shampoo treatments in the form of lightweight masks (a cream-gel formula can be good for you); the excess will be washed out when you shampoo.

Volume may well be top of your hairstyling wish list; nowadays, there are fantastic volumising ranges that really do add body, bounce and root-lift. Try one of the very affordable, mainstream ranges now available on the high street first; if that doesn't give the volume you want, trade up to a pricier version. You wear your hair every day; I'd say it's worth investing in it. I wouldn't mix-and-match; volumising ranges are trialled as regimes and you'll almost certainly get the best results from using the products across a single range.

Product-wise, fine hair responds better to mousses, powders, water-based serums and gels, as well as dry shampoos. These are definitely not just for getting hair clean; they're brilliant for adding guts to fine hair. When hair is towel-dry, you can add a volumising spray to the roots and a water-based primer or serum to the lengths to plump up each hair strand.

And remember: one of the best tricks for fine hair is always to dry it upside-down, to get air and volume into the roots.

MEDIUM HAIR

Like 'normal' skin, medium-textured hair is something you can count your blessings for. Hair isn't thin, or thick: it's somewhere in between. You have your pick of suits-all-hair types products, so it's really down to the effect you want. Do you long for extra volume? Or more gloss and sleekness and an ultra-smooth finish? Products which deliver those results will all work on your hair texture. Your hair is probably also pretty resilient to styling, but mask treatments once a week are definitely recommended. Your hair can also take rich conditioning treatments, especially when you want to create a slick style.

THICK HAIR

When you have thick hair, that doesn't necessarily mean you've more follicles on your scalp (though that may also be the case); it's really referring to the thickness or courseness of the individual hair strands. With thick hair, you can really feel the individual strands and fibres of the hair, and when it's healthy, it's wonderfully strong hair. But thick hair is thirsty hair: quite simply, there's more surface area and so the cuticle (semi-circular layers on the outside of the strand, invisible to the naked eye) can lift up, causing dryness. So thick hair responds to serums, oils, creams and pomades, with regular deep conditioning treatments to keep it shiny and supple. Use pre-shampoo oil treatments, but also masks that are slathered onto wet hair and rinsed out like a conditioner, which will inevitably leave some of the oil to protect the strands. With styling products, the richer the texture the better, but you may find that you get through product fast, in order to get the results you want.

Alison's Tip ——————————————————

Hair health changes as the seasons change, so keep re-evaluating your products, shade and style.

CURLY/WAVY HAIR

Curls or waves happen with all different hair structures – fine, medium, thick. A curl emerges from a twisted follicle, and continues to twist as it grows, which means that the cuticles on the surface lift up. This can make the hair prone to dryness and vulnerable to breakage and split ends, especially as a result of rough treatment or other damage.

When you're getting your hair cut, ask for the hairdresser at any given salon who's great at dealing with curly hair. If you've tight curls, go to someone who specialises in Afro hair, because they'll give you the best cut.

As for at-home care, the thicker and wirier your hair, the less often you'll need to wash it. Thick, curly hair actually responds to *not* washing as the natural oils tame curls: you might get away with every two or three days, or even two weeks between washes, depending on whether you live in a polluted town or city, or the country and depending, too, on how clean you like your scalp to feel. But if you've habitually washed your hair frequently, experiment with extending the time between shampoos.

There are many regimes now specifically for curly and wavy hair. If you like to straighten your hair, you need serums or styling products which trumpet the fact they offer 'heat protection'. Use the diffuser attachment on your hairdryer and also check out the modern jet-streaming driers, which dry quickly, without causing frizz. If you're using straightening tools, always blow-dry first, before using flattening irons, and use heat-protecting styling products or a serum, first.

Daily moisturising is needed to keep hair luscious, in the form of styling creams or oils, smoothed into straightened hair or scrunched into curls with damp hands.

Weekly moisturising hair masks are a must, whether or not you use heat to style. They're not designed for application to the scalp; the hair furthest from your scalp is the oldest, and needs the most lavish treatment. There are many different mask options now: some you put on before you shower, some you can sleep in. Generally with masks, the longer you can leave them on the hair, the better the results you'll get. You may even be able to scrunch a mask into curls and leave it there between washes, if you really need added moisture. And more is more is more.

TO GO GREY – OR NOT TO GO GREY...?
THAT IS THE QUESTION

The brilliant news about grey hair is that it's not necessarily ageing any longer. It's now a massive fashion statement, embraced by everyone from teens upwards, who are crazy for violet, grey, indigo and purple rinses. Grey can also be hugely flattering, as well as being massively more low-maintenance than colouring your hair. Overall, you'll be saving lots of money and hassle, because colouring roots and regrowth need to be dealt with on a constant, ongoing basis, as often as every two weeks, if you have brunette or black hair. That's a lot of upkeep. Just look around: in print media, on TV and across social media, you'll find actors, models and public figures all embracing the grey – and don't they look wonderful...?

If you've always had very dark hair and a pale complexion, there comes a point when it no longer flatters to dye your hair dark. But whatever colour your hair is now – dyed or natural – the best path towards embracing the grey is with the help of your hair colourist/stylist. If you had paler hair before, grey or white isn't a huge leap from where you were anyway, in terms of your colouring. If hair is becoming naturally salt and pepper as it grows out, a hairdresser can give you advice on how to manage this, perhaps with a shorter cut. If you've always had dark hair, they may suggest gradually lightening it, so the grey is almost blurred, rather than obvious regrowth. Or go blonde for the first time; it's easier maintenance as regrowth isn't so obvious.

Another reason behind the growing numbers embracing their grey is that the products designed to care for grey hair have made great technological leaps forward. Even 20 years ago, grey hair tended to look coarse, and could be prone to yellowing. Nowadays, thanks to sleeking serums and products to counterbalance any yellow, grey can look smooth and vibrant. Detox shampoos can take out unwanted pollution, while violet-toned shampoos or blue masks counterbalance any 'brassiness'. Add in a shine serum, and you can look head-turningly fabulous.

Your make-up may need adjusting as you embrace the grey. You may find that make-up becomes much easier: your eyes may pop more

TO WASH OR NOT TO WASH?

Don't get in a lather over whether or not to wash your hair daily. The longer you can leave your hair between washes, while still ensuring it looks good, the better for it. If you're a daily shampooer, try a few weeks of every other day. You may be surprised by how positively it responds – and you'll definitely love the extra time it's given you back into what's almost certainly a busy life. Pop on a shower cap to extend the time between washes. I hadn't owned a shower cap for decades, but they've come right back in and are infinitely more efficient than before. The exception is if you work in the medical world or food preparation (hair absorbs food smells very easily), or do a lot of sport; if it leaves you sweaty, you may want to wash daily. If this is you, or you wish to wash daily, choose a frequent wash product/regime.

and your complexion looks healthier, because dark hair can pick out the shadows on a face. Conversely, you may find that you look a bit more washed-out and need some extra help in the form of blusher and brow colour, to give your face structure. (Strong spectacle frames can be very stylish with grey and white hair, too.) This really is the time to open up your 'Make-up Toybox' (see p. 151) and play with products. You may find that – like many a chic Frenchwoman – you can now reach for a red lipstick, and that's all you need to look striking with your grey hair. But whatever make-up look you settle on, make the most of the opportunity to reinvent yourself and become a whole new you.

Love your scalp

G reat hair starts with a healthy scalp, so start taking a more skincare-led approach to this oft-overlooked part of our bodies…

There's a buzz about the scalp in the beauty world, and quite rightly, because it's literally at the root of great-looking hair.

It would be easy to take an 'out-of-sight, out-of-mind' approach to the scalp – it's largely hidden for many of us. But in fact, the scalp is unique, and deserves some special care. With the density of hair follicles, high rate of oil production and the heat factor, many of us suffer from scalp sweating, even without hoods and hats.; these all combine to affect the scalp's natural microbiome, or its balance of yeast and bacteria. Happily, there's a much better understanding today of what the scalp needs to be healthy, and technologies and ingredients are advancing all the time.

Each hair emerges from (and grows through) an individual follicle on the scalp. That follicle also produces sebum (oil), and as we pass through the stages of life, the amount of oil will vary. If the follicles become blocked by sebum or dead skin, this can lead to scalp problems (and there's a risk that permanently blocked or obstructed follicles may cease to produce hair at all). The scalp itself is made up of cells which continually work their way to the surface, and those need removing, and not just by washing and brushing. This skin around the hair can also suffer from condition and ageing concerns.

Scalp troubles that affect both men and women include itching, flaking, oiliness and dandruff, but you needn't put up with any of these nowadays. The scalp may also be affected by eczema, psoriasis and other dermatological problems, about which you may need to talk to a medical professional; your doctor may refer you to a dermatologist or a trichologist (a specialist in hair and the scalp). If your skin is dry, your scalp – an extension of your face – may well be dry too.

Even if your scalp's perfectly well-behaved, it's worth remembering that all good hair days begin with a healthy scalp. Here's what you can do to help:

- **A healthy scalp begins with a balanced diet.**
  With our incredibly busy lives, it can be difficult to guarantee that we get the full range of nutrients every single day, so do consider taking a hair/nails/skin supplement as a sort of nutritional 'insurance policy'. Look for a brand that's been around for many years, or perhaps which specialises in researching hair and scalp health.

- **Scrub your scalp.**
  Just like the skin on the body, flakes build up on the scalp. A lot of specific scalp exfoliators are appearing on the market now, but for general scalp health you can also use the regular salt or jojoba-based exfoliator that you'd normally use on your body, working it into the scalp area and rinsing well. It's likely to be an oil-based product, so do this before your first shampoo; the oils, however, will ensure that the scalp isn't over-stripped.

- **Mud's great for oily scalps.**
  Mud (rhassoul mud from Morocco, or any kind of clay/kaolin) is brilliant for tackling oil and grease and removing toxins. Massage a mud-based mask into the scalp weekly, to get the

CHECK THE LABELS

Two particularly common shampoo ingredients, Sodium Lauryl Sulfate (SLS) and Sodium Laureth Sulfate (SLES), are linked with scalp sensitivity and itching, so screen your products for this and if you're experiencing an itchy scalp, switch to an SLS/SLES-free product. These are ever-more-widely available – you may even find that your favourite mainstream shampoo brand is now available SLS-free. Natural stores often have a particularly good selection.

benefit of its oil-reducing, flake-eliminating effects. You can shop your beauty cabinet for this: if you use a mud mask on your face, have a go with that rather than buying a specific hair mud; beauty products are much more multitasking than manufacturers would have us think!

- **If you have a dry or itchy scalp, try an oil treatment.**
While oily scalps respond well to mud, the answer for a dry scalp is an oil treatment. Again, there are many dedicated scalp oils appearing on the market, but you can use the inexpensive single oil that you might have for use on your face, and which you know you're not sensitive to. Massage about a tablespoonful into your fingertips and massage onto the scalp, working into the scalp and the roots of the hair to soften and loosen dry skin before washing. Leave it on for 10–15 minutes before shampooing and conditioning as normal. Repeat weekly (or if your scalp is very dry, do this before each wash).

- **Try a scalp-soother.**
Use the cooling jelly inside the leaf of an aloe plant, mashed with a fork and applied to the scalp as a weekly pre-shampoo mask treatment. (Alternatively, use an aloe vera gel from a natural food store.) You can also drench cotton wool pads in witch hazel or a simple flower water (lavender/orange flower) and swab the scalp. Or check out one of the specific scalp-soothing lotions or drizzles, some of which feature probiotics or prebiotics to balance the scalp's microbiome. (The ones with nozzles or droppers make application easier.)

Alison's Tip

If you have a spotty back, forehead or chest, avoid the 'waterfall' of shampoo and conditioner running over your skin when in the shower as the ingredients may be causing the problem. Alternatively, change to an SLS-free or 'free-from' formula.

- **Check out detoxing shampoos.**

Sometimes also referred to as 'clarifying' shampoos, these are specifically formulated to eliminate build-up from styling products and/or city pollution, while rebalancing and nourishing the scalp. They're also good if you work out, as natural oils and sweat can unbalance even the happiest scalp. Once upon a time these detoxing products were very drying, but that's starting to change. You can also find natural and 'free-from' formulas. You don't need to have an itchy, oily or inflamed scalp to use a detoxing shampoo – they can be a valuable addition to your haircare 'wardrobe', for occasional use.

- **Don't get burned.**

The scalp is very vulnerable to sunburn, particularly for anyone who has thinning hair, wears their hair with a parting, or has braids and corn-rows. My No.1 prevention from burning is shade. A hat does the job, or sitting under a parasol or in the shade of a tree or awning. You can also buy sun protection (serums/creams) specifically for the hair and scalp, often in spritz-on format, for ease.

- **Avoid heat damage during styling.**

Some hairdryers really blast out very intense heat, which is drying and damaging (almost burning) to the scalp, and will definitely make the problem worse, if you've a tendency to dryness. Keep hairdryer use to a minimum, if you have any scalp problems. Instead, gently towel-dry hair till it's roughly 80 per cent dry, then apply styling products and finish with a hairdryer. Look for hairdryers with smart tech, like ionic and 'airflow' dryers, which are becoming more affordable and dry hair quicker without excess heat.

- **Shampoo skills.**

Most people shampoo using the flat of the hand, which means that you never really clarify the scalp and roots. Instead, use a strong fingertip massage to get the suds to the scalp. If you've long or thick hair, lift up sections to get the foam underneath onto the root area. Also do this to aim the spray of the shower water.

Alison's Tip ───────────────────────────────

Hair holds fragrance incredibly well, so it's a fantastic place to spray scent. A zoosh of a gorgeous scent can be a godsend when your hair's picked up smells from cooking, or perhaps a bonfire. But don't just use your regular perfume, which may be too alcoholic and drying. Many well-loved perfume ranges now offer fragrances which are specifically formulated for spritzing onto hair itself. If you don't have a hair fragrance, alternatively, you can lift up the back of your hair and spray your usual scent on the nape of the neck, where it will waft beautifully.

Ask Alison: hair Q&A

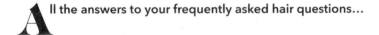

All the answers to your frequently asked hair questions…

Q: How do I get volume in my hair?

First of all, thank your lucky stars to be styling your hair in the 2020s: volumising products are better than they have ever been! You can now buy ranges which are specifically for creating volume – shampoo, conditioner, styling products, plumping serum, root-lift spray and mousse. Use a system from one hair brand, as these will have been trialled together for the best results. Hairdresser brand 'systems' are amazing at this. You'll notice the difference; bigger hair can even balance out an outfit.

   With styling products, a little can go a long way; you'll need to play around to discover which creates the optimum fullness in your hair. But technique plays a part, too. Blow-dry your hair upside-down, or against the way it's going to fall, until the final stages, as this gets more lift into the root area. Velcro or heated rollers on the crown can also help; leave them there until the hair cools down, or for as long as you like, actually; just remove them when you need to.

Dry shampoos and volume-blast products are also your friends; volume-blast products are like a cross between hair spray and a dry shampoo, rather like a 'backcomb in a can'. They're great for flat fringes or a flat crown when you get up in the morning, to save you having to restyle your hair.

Q: What can I do about curls that drop right out again?

If you have naturally curly hair, curl-enhancing products are your go-to here, specifically designed to define curls and keep the natural shape for longer, preventing frizziness. Spritz a curl-enhancing spray onto your hair and let it dry naturally, wrapping around your fingers for shape. Then if you want more definition, curl it with a curling tong/wand. If you're trying to encourage a curl in straight hair, primers and styling serums are essential, as are hair sprays. If they have heat protection built in spray before heat styling, as well as after. Use tongs to create curl and pin the curls in place with hair pins, or use heated rollers. Leave the rollers or pinned curls in place for as long as possible to encourage the wave or curl to stay; you may want to style your hair before you do your make-up and get ready, then finger separate or shake out the curls at the end. Spritzing with hairspray is optional, depending on whether you like the effect it gives.

Q: How can I make my hairstyle last for a special occasion?

First off: don't wash it on the day itself; hair needs some natural oils in order to keep a style. Wash and get a great blow dry the day before, or if you have very curly or afro hair, it's fine to wash it two or three days beforehand, so the natural oils have time to come through. Natural oils are essential for grip, as freshly washed hair is sleek and slippery. If you're adding a hairpiece, backcombing or using hair accessories, these will all stay put better if hair isn't squeaky-clean. Dry shampoo spritzed into hair can also be useful to add guts, body, grip and staying power, before styling.

If you're having your hair done professionally, tell them what time your big event is (e.g. that afternoon or evening), and they'll create something that will look its very best at that time. If you're doing your hair yourself, experiment in advance with heated or Velcro rollers, tonging or pin-curling to get the fullness you want. Nowadays, you can get great, natural-looking hold from hairsprays – shop around for one that doesn't give you 'helmet-hair', and it will also help your style to last.

Q: Is it safe to backcomb?

The only time I'd ever advise backcombing is for a very special event, and even then, I think it's best left to professionals (i.e. your hairdresser). Backcombing is definitely damaging on an ongoing basis, because it pushes the cuticle open, going against the grain, encouraging breakage and splitting high up the hair shaft.

You can avoid the need for backcombing now with root-lift/volumising products and drying your hair upside-down (see p.239). Alternatively, you can invest in a thin hair crimper: use to crimp just the first inch of hair; not around the parting or hairline, which would be too obvious, but the hair underneath, to add invisible lift. If you do decide to backcomb, be ready with plenty of conditioner or detangling spray to comb through afterwards.

Q: I know I should use a hair mask but won't it make my hair greasy?

Look for a pre-shampoo mask and treatment, so that any excess is shampooed out. Choose a cream-gel or a moisture-rich, lightweight mask. If you're prone to greasiness from heavy conditioners, these lighter masks are a revelation and a great way of adding extra gloss and condition to hair that's prone to oiliness.

Split hair, like split nails, can be sealed with a product. |

Q: What can I do about split ends?

Gone are the days when you had to chop these off! Split hair, like split nails, can be sealed with a product. Split ends happen because of a natural process. If you were to look at hair under a microscope you'd see that every hair is covered with little semi-circular overlapping cuticles, which lift up when they become dry or brittle. You can close these down again with moisturising products, hair masks and serums; specific 'split end' products work a bit like a sticking plaster on the split end itself. So unless the ends of your hair have become very ratty because these cuticles have sheared off, a split end sealant, hair serum or lotion can be your greatest hairstyling allies; these smooth down the cuticle and make your hair thicker down the whole length of the strand, as well as the ends.

Curly hair is more prone to split ends because of the way the cortex of the hair twists, which encourages lifting of the cuticles. Moisturising products and masks are even more important. Between washes, boost moisture via a dab or two of conditioner smoothed into palms and scrunched into hair.

Just one more command (and I'm going to be bossy, here): Never. Pull. Split. Ends. Apart. (Ever.) You will make the hair thinner and it can never be truly healed.

Q: Do extensions damage my hair?

Clip-in inserts or bonded hair extensions can be great short-term solutions, offering a confidence-boost, or if you want a certain style for a special occasion. The downside with professionally bonded hair extensions is that if you come to depend on them, they will cause tension and eventually breakage where they've been attached to your natural hair. It's also easy to become psychologically dependent on them, with confidence taking quite a dip when they're removed.

Clip-in extensions can be easily put in and taken out for big dates and special occasions; they're not expensive and come in really realistic shades. They come as individual clip-in extensions which you attach in a semi-circle from one side of your head to the other, and are then disguised under the top layer of hair. (Your regular hairdresser may be happy to advise on how best to use them.) Used too regularly, though, even these can be damaging where the clip clamps onto the hair.

Q: How can I manage my textured curls?

There are several different categories of coils and curls, but most respond to less frequent washing. Once a week, once a fortnight, or even less frequently than that, can be helpful. In between, you want to lavish your hair with oils, butters and heavier-weight moisturising masks. As often as every day, introduce moisture into the ends of your hair by smooshing conditioner or spray hydrators between your palms, then scrunching into the ends of the curls, which you can wind around your finger to refresh at the same time. If you have a smoother style, meanwhile, or gentler waves, you can brush oils through from root to ends with bristle-type brushes. With your hair, the mantra for product is: more is more is more.

Because textured hair is very porous, it can take up to four or five hours to dry naturally. A modern hairdryer – always with a diffuser and a low heat setting – can speed things up somewhat, but be aware always that your hair is actually quite fragile and can tear very easily. However you manage it, do it with lashings of TLC.

Q: How do I use dry shampoo?

These are for use on dry hair, not hair that's wet from shampooing. Dry shampoos are great for refreshing your hair after a workout, after sport, when you've cycled to work, at menopause or anytime the scalp gets sweaty, because the powder in the shampoo is absorbent.

As far as the how-to goes, first shake your can to mix the liquid/powder and any fibre elements inside, otherwise what comes out of the nozzle will just be a whoosh of wetness. Lift up sections of the hair all over the head, including at the crown and the fringe, giving a burst of dry shampoo into the roots. If you have longer hair, you can tip your hair upside down and spritz the shampoo into sections of the roots.

If it's cleanliness you're after, brush through after a minute or two, and the oils from your hair will be removed by this brushing. If it's volume you want, work the dry shampoo into the roots and massage the scalp with fingertips, for instant oomph.

Q: How can I make my greasy hair less lank?

Dry shampoo, again (see above). They're the be-all and end-all of modern styling and hair troubleshooting. You can also do a weekly mud deep cleanse to absorb excess oil and aerate the scalp.

Q: How can I prevent breakage from braiding?

Braiding can pull and tug at the roots of hair, leading to hair snapping off almost at scalp level. If breakage is becoming a problem, sometimes changing the direction of how your style falls can help. Next time you have your braids done, ask if they can be created with less tension at the root and with less hair in each braid to reduce weight. Maybe don't have them done so often; there's a movement towards embracing natural hair, but another alternative is a wig, if you don't want to go *au naturel*.

If you're a regular braider consider using scalp drops powered by minerals and vitamins to help with hair strength and health, and laser treatments that stimulate the root.

Q: What's the best way to detangle hair?

Try to avoid clothing that tangles hair, such as woolly scarves; if you're going for a blustery walk tie hair up so it can't whip around. Some hair types are more prone to tangling: very fine or very curly hair, hair that is coloured or just dry. If your hair tends to tangle, trade up to a stronger conditioner and use it as a weekly mask.

If you're prone to this, every time you wash use a detangling spray, serum or a touch of oil, combed through from end to root; start with a wide-toothed comb (never a normal comb) or specific wet hair detangler at the ends of hair first, gradually working up towards the root to detangle as you go, rather than starting at the top and moving down.

In between washes, spritz on a daily hydrating leave-in conditioner/mist; if you don't want to spray this directly onto the hair, spritz it onto a vent brush or a wide-toothed comb instead and brush that through. Frizz and tangling in the night can also be helped by switching to a silk pillowcase.

If your child has hair that tangles, be aware that you may need to treat them to specific haircare that's different to the rest of the family, in order to get the knots out without hurting. A leave-in conditioner can be really helpful, while you get the tangles out of a child's hair. A spray or serum used afterwards will help prevent hair reknotting each day.

Q: What's the best way to manage frizzy hair?

If your hair goes frizzy between washes, anti-frizz moisturising sprays are your go-to. It's all about adding extra condition, whenever possible. These can also be used to refresh your style or rework your fringe, without the need to start from scratch. (They often smell quite lovely, as a bonus.)

If your hair has been in a damp and humid environment, put some of your regular conditioner into the palm of your hand, and add just a little water before scrunching into your hair to smooth and reactivate the curl, taking away the frizz.

Ionic hairdryers and air dryers really do make a difference for you, because they stop hair being over-dried at high temperature. Do also look out for hairbrushes with an 'anti-frizz' coating or battery operated ionising function.

Take an umbrella and bucket hat or a headscarf with you to cover up the minute the weather turns drizzly. Fine rain can get underneath umbrellas and turn you frizzy.

Alison's Tip

Don't be shy to take your own shampoo and conditioner to the salon and ask them to use it, if you feel the range of products they carry impact negatively on your hair colour. I can promise you that every beauty editor in the country arrives at a salon armed with their own haircare!

Q: How can I make my colour last?

Colour-enhancing shampoos, conditioners and masks are designed exactly for this and come in all shade options, so if you colour your hair, you need to buy products to help protect it. Some of them actually add a little colour back into the hair, while others simply work to keep the colour bright and vibrant. Violet-toned shampoos, for instance, work to counterbalance the yellowing that blonde hair can develop. Colour care shampoos, conditioners and masks may be free of colour, but again, are formulated with ingredients to keep your colour vibrant and make it last. These formulas will almost always be free of SLS/SLES (Sodium Lauryl/ Laureth Sulfate), which are detergents that can lift colour from hair.

If you're headed to your colourist for a salon colour (or colouring your hair at home) use a detox shampoo first. This will help ensure that your base hair colour is more 'true', and in the case of salon colouring, will help the hairdresser to assess which products will deliver the result you want. If your chosen hair colour is a pale shade, you may also want to use a detox shampoo every couple of weeks, to remove pollutants that can build up and affect your chosen colour.

Q: Will regular saunas damage my hair?

On the contrary, they can be great for hair; this is the perfect moment for a scalp oil treatment, a mask, a mud mask… The heat will encourage penetration, though to avoid mess, do wrap your hair in an (unprecious) towel when you go in. Afterwards, shampoo and condition as normal. This is the equivalent of an expensive thalassotherapy hotel spa treatment – so make the most of it!

Q: My hair's being damaged because of my bike helmet/visor – what can I do?

When you first get it fitted, do so with your hair in the style you will usually wear it, so it's safe and comfortable. Adjust the visor/helmet so that when you put it on, there are absolutely no pulls and tugs that can cause breakage; it's worth taking a couple of minutes to adjust the position of the helmet/visor each time, to avoid friction and pulling, and to ensure that there's no hair trapped in Velcro fastenings or clips.

If you still find that there's tugging or that the fastenings are rubbing the scalp, massage moisturiser or a simple base oil (almond, coconut or argan) into the skin regularly, to nourish and condition it.

If you cycle/bike regularly, tuck your hair inside your helmet where possible to reduce weather damage.

Q: How can I prevent my hair from getting damaged when I swim?

Wet your hair before you go into the pool and smooth in a hair mask or conditioner. When your hair is damp from the shower, it means the hair cuticle has swelled, which stops it from filling up with chlorine, which can both dry hair and give it a green or turquoise tone. The mask or conditioner will also nourish and protect the hair; rinse or shampoo it out after swimming (and if the latter, condition again).

Love your body

"

Life is too short to be hung up on 'flaws' and 'imperfections'

We only have one body. And one life. It's much too short to be hung up on 'flaws' and 'imperfections', so here's how to feel more comfortable in the skin you're in. (Literally.)

Something I've observed time and again is that for many people, their beauty regime stops at the jawline. It's as if the rest of the body doesn't exist. But giving yourself plenty of TLC from neck to toe is really important. The skin is the largest organ of the body so we owe it to ourselves to look after it.

It upsets me when I hear people 'hate' this or that about their bodies. When I look at someone, I don't see their size and shape. I'm taking in the fact they're stylishly dressed, or look warm and friendly, or have a great smile. Try to surround yourself with people who give you positive reinforcement rather than being critical. A friend who is critical isn't a real friend at all.

We can't freeze-frame ourselves at the age of 18 or 30; we all have 'badges of life' in the form of scars, stretch marks, or wrinkles. What we can do is look after the body we do have, to the best of our ability.

Connecting with your body in a mindful way, using beautiful products with gorgeous scents and textures, is a way of being kind to yourself. Sometimes just the fragrance of a product is enough to lift your spirits and make you smile.

When it comes to body care, I do think it helps to 'accentuate the positive' – most of us have bits we feel good about: nice hands or feet, an attractive décolletage, lovely eyes, great hair... If you draw attention to the parts of your body you're happiest with, I promise you that nobody, but nobody, is going to notice the thread vein on your knee that bothers you.

There's a lot of simple, inexpensive or even free stuff that we can do on a regular basis to improve things: from body-brushing, drinking water and stretching that boost our body self-care. In a world in which we live in our heads so much of the time – thinking, thinking, thinking – it can feel very grounding to give some attention to the body, as a way of reconnecting with the rest of ourselves.

So, take your time over this chapter, and find new ways to show yourself some wonderful self-care.

Body basics

This is where everyone should start with their body self-care. If you want to add steps and products into your ritual, that's entirely up to you, but these are the essentials that we all need to do:

Priority 1: Washing

This is the most important part of our body care routine and if you choose your products well, you may not need to use a body moisturiser. The key is to make sure you're washing with something which doesn't leave it drier than before.

If you're shopping for bar soap, seek out one that has a high oil content, for instance, a base of olive oil or shea butters. Ideally, choose one with glycerine, too, which works to attract moisture to the skin. This means it will be less drying.

If you're using a shower gel or any foaming body product, choose one with some oil in there. Check out the new generation of shower oils, which leave skin nourished while getting it perfectly clean; incorporating natural oils like sweet almond, jojoba or grapeseed oil, they emulsify and turn into a rich milk foam on contact with water, leaving skin satiny

If you have sensitive skin, irritation or rashes, avoid the ingredients SLS/SLES (Sodium Lauryl Sulfate/Sodium Laureth Sulfate), as these can dry the skin and leave it irritated. It can help to look for products with a short ingredients list; there's less in there to cause a reaction. (Although with any body product, I still always recommend a patch test before first use – see tip below)

Alison's Tip

To body patch test, apply a little of the new product to a delicate area of the body such as the inside of the arm (the crook of the elbow is ideal), or a small part of the area you're planning to use it on. Check 24 hours later for signs of irritation, redness or itching. If there are no adverse reactions, you're good to go. Technically you should do this with every new product: body oil, shower gel, body wash, body lotion, exfoliator – and you should certainly do so if you have reactive skin.

Priority 2: Exfoliation.

It doesn't matter how great your body moisturiser is, if your skin's covered in dry, dead cells, it's not going to be able to do its job properly – anything you put on it will just sit on the surface. I'd have everyone (except sufferers of psoriasis or eczema) exfoliating their body twice a week, because it can make such a massive difference to skin softness.

You can exfoliate by skin brushing (see p.257) or use a body scrub or enzymatic exfoliator. Apply oil-based and cream-based exfoliators before bathing, when you'll get the strongest action. If you have more sensitive skin, use them on wet skin in the bath or shower.

Some salt and sugar scrubs are suspended in oil, which can be good for two reasons: if you use one of these scrubs before the bath, the salt or sugar will dissolve and the oil will disperse into the water so as you emerge from your bath a veil of scented nourishment will be left on the surface of skin as the oil clings to it.

These scrubs can also double up as hand scrubs if you tend to get grubby hands from work, gardening or DIY, for instance. (What I would add, though, is that if you tend to get scratched for any reason, then go for the sugar scrub, because otherwise you may find yourself literally rubbing salt into an open wound.)

If you use a grainy, gritty scrub, perhaps with skin-buffing particles of nuts or pumice, then I recommend using these in the shower, otherwise you can end up sitting in a bath with a very uncomfortably gritty bottom – not at all the soothing, sensual experience that we generally want a bath to be.

Chemical/enzymatic exfoliants work by gently dissolving the top layers of skin that are dead and ready to be removed. These often come in the form of a body lotion, perhaps infused with AHAs (such as glycolic acid, see Ingredients, p.114), and some may even have a bit of glow or shimmer in there. The action is subtler than a physical scrub and you'll need to apply daily; these products work their magic while sitting on the skin's surface, so unlike scrubs, you don't wash them off.

Priority 3: Putting back the moisture.

Simple rule of thumb here: the drier your skin, the richer your body lotion should be and the more often you should apply it. If your skin is really dry and feels tight or uncomfortable, you'll probably find an oil is best for you and it will be a daily (or rather, nightly) must.

If you have a dark skin tone, you may find that your skin becomes ashy-looking; this is simply a result of dry surface skin cells contrasted against the natural colour of your skin. The answer is to use a body butter or an oil daily, which will not only deliver a surge of moisture but also instant comfort and glow. Oils are best used before bedtime because they can make it a little sticky. I like to apply oils to damp skin, after I've showered or bathed. Butters are easier to apply on dry skin.

Many people find they don't need to reach for body lotion or cream every day, especially if you've chosen a non-drying body cleansing product. Dry body skin often doesn't become a problem for many

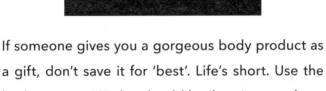

EVERY DAY IS 'BEST'

If someone gives you a gorgeous body product as a gift, don't save it for 'best'. Life's short. Use the body cream...! Today should be 'best', every day – and besides, products don't have an infinite shelf life, so use them sooner rather than later.

people until their 40s. For you, a body product might be something fragrant that you put on for special occasions. A lot of people only really bother with a body routine when a holiday's looming and they realise it needs to be show-offable. In that case, it's your preference as to whether you use a lotion, cream, butter or oil.

Any face cream will also work as a body cream. So if you've got a face product that isn't doing what you want it to, don't throw it away or leave it languishing in your cupboard: stick it on your bedside table and use it on your body instead.

If your skin's going to be exposed to UV, you need a body product with an SPF, to be worn on a daily basis. Make sure the tops of the hands and feet are protected, and any other bits that are going to be on show.

Alison's Tip

My bedside table has an array of products on it for night-time use (and sometimes again in the morning). If you can see your lotions and potions, you'll be reminded to use them diligently. I've always got an aromatherapy product for sleep – an inhalation or oil; a hand and a foot treatment; lip balm (I put this on very last thing at night); lip serum for the lines between lips and nose; body cream or butter; and last but not least, a facial moisturiser that can be used on face, neck and eyes if I wake up with tight, dry skin. If you're trying to work on an area, such as under the eyes, then put your product for this on your bedside table too and reapply as often as you can.

Body brush how-to

The quickest, easiest and cheapest way to improve body tone and the softness of skin is to body brush. It's up to you whether you use a long-handled brush or a brush that fits in the palm of your hand, but when you're brush-shopping, run the brush over the back of the hand to try it out – if it leaves visible scratch-marks (usually just fine white lines of dead skin), it's too hard. You want something that has softish bristles, and you'll find that it will still exfoliate effectively. Brushing boosts circulation, improves glow and skin condition and gently exfoliates the surface so that body products sink in more effectively. You're stimulating the largest organ of the body and it leaves you feeling tingling and alive, so I'd be surprised if you don't get a little addicted once you try it.

1   Start at one ankle, sweeping up the leg, a few sweeps all over the lower legs and thighs. Then the other leg. Body-brushing is a brilliant cellulite treatment, because it moves the lymph and disperses toxins, while bringing nutrients to the skin. Sweep the brush over each buttock, always upwards.

2   Move on to brush the arms, starting at the wrist and moving towards the shoulders, again, a few sweeps each time. Repeat on the other arm.

3   Always move towards the heart in an upwards direction, rather than to-and-fro.

4   Ideally, body brush once a day. Before showering or bathing is the ideal time, but you should always do it on dry skin, rather than wetted skin. If you feel you don't have time every day, carve out a few minutes a couple of times a week, or put it next to your bed and do it just before bedtime.

5   Newly brushed skin should be moisturised, either following your bath or shower, or straight after brushing if you're not bathing or showering.

BODY TROUBLESHOOTING

How to answer an S.O.S. from body skin and make it all bareable again…

For most of us, a regular body regime keeps problems at bay. But when things flare up, it can be puzzling and often downright distressing. In some cases, you'll need to see your doctor, but very often, at-home solutions can transform how the skin on your body looks and, just as importantly, feels.

Slack body skin

Nobody gets to have firm, plumptious, resilient skin forever. Slackened skin is a sign of body ageing, and it'll happen to all of us. Some things do speed it up: gaining and losing weight, puffing up with fluid, pregnancy. It's a fact of life, inescapable – but that doesn't mean there aren't some clever fixes:

- Exfoliate your skin three times a week (see p.253).

- Use a body brush daily to invigorate skin; it'll improve blood circulation, smooth away lymph and fluid and make skin more receptive to products.

- Choose a body moisturiser with firming ingredients.

- Use self-tanner, whatever your skin tone. It makes everyone's skin look better (and if you use a tinted product, you'll see an instant transformation).

Stretch marks

Oh, I've seen thousands of these, over the years, when giving treatments. Women will almost always get them at some point, to a greater or lesser degree, but men can get stretch marks too. I don't think they're anything to feel self-conscious about – but so many people are. Stretch marks happen when the body expands because of weight/growth, and they have a hormonal link, too – sometimes oestrogen, sometimes (more often in men) cortisol production.

The time we most often associate with stretch marks is pregnancy, but they can often happen at puberty. Weight gain can result in stretch marks, but it's actually the hormonal changes triggered by putting on weight that causes the stretch marks. Sometimes, they just show up for no apparent reason at all.

A stretch mark 'breaks' deep in the dermis, before it's visible. When stretch marks first make their way to the surface, the epidermis, they're often red or burgundy in colour. Over time, they fade to pale, silvery streaks.

You may not be able to stop them appearing, but you can ensure that skin is as supple as it can be. Even when you're planning a pregnancy, and certainly once it's confirmed, slather skin with rich moisturisers, oils and butters on a daily basis. The tummy isn't the only area that can be affected; they can crop up from knee to neck, front and back, so include the whole body in your daily massage routine. Sometimes you'll get them early on but sometimes it isn't till the fifth or sixth month that they start to show up, so keep moisturising even if nothing has appeared yet.

You can't get rid of stretch marks, but you can lessen their appearance with gentle scrubs and lotions. If your stretch marks are recent, don't sunbathe – in fact, don't sunbathe till a stretch mark is at least a year old, because that will prevent them thickening and pigmenting.

There are several ways to disguise stretch marks, if you feel self-conscious:

- Self-tan can be your easy go-to; treat it like semi-permanent body make-up, to even up your skin tone.

- Use a body foundation; these are water-resistant, so you can swim in them and they have a surprisingly plumping, conditioning action.

- There are more opaque, dense cosmetic forms of body make-up designed to conceal scarring if you really feel you need to disguise your marks. They come in different shades and nowadays are easy to find online; the skin tone of the models photographed is honestly a really good guide to the tint you'll get, so match yours to the photos.

- There are salon procedures such as chemical peels and laser therapy, designed to reduce the appearance of stretch marks. Ask to see actual real-life client photos, not just promotional materials, before you take one of these options. Be aware that no treatment can banish them completely.

- My best advice is to try to relax about stretch marks and accept them as another of those 'badges of life' which make us who we are – and that's OK.

Body odour

We all have body odour; it's natural. It's caused by our natural excretory process; it's how the body gets rid of toxins, with sweat coming out through sweat glands and pores all over the face, scalp and body, not just the underarms or the genital area.

If you're exercising, it's definitely very good for sweat to come out in the underarm area, so don't try to stop it with antiperspirants, which work to block the pores. You want that sweat, those toxins, out of there. In a work or social setting, you may want to use an anti-perspirant to avoid visible wetness, but you can often make a big difference to body odour by switching to an antiseptic body wash or adding in a couple of drops of tea tree oil to your regular body cleanser.

Some people are naturally more prone to sweating, which can become odorous when bacteria go into overdrive and your natural body flora/microbiome is out of whack. You can easily have a situation where you shower, yet within half an hour, your armpits are whiffy again. Adding in an antibacterial/tea tree wash to your regime may help. Leave the foam on your skin for several minutes before washing it off.

Others develop body odour after an illness like 'flu, as a result of medication, during menopause, because of stresses like job interviews or exams. If you're suffering from really excessive sweating, this can be an indication that you need to see a doctor.

I'm all too familiar with sweating; as a teen at school, I often couldn't take off my jumper because the patches on my school shirt were so large they met in the middle. These days, I drive an HGV and a tractor, I appear on live television, and I'm menopausal – trust me, I still sweat. If I didn't follow my own advice (below), I'd still suffer from body odour. Here's what to do:

- The temptation is to spray all over with a strong antiperspirant and/or deodorant to 'block' the sweat. But these block your natural excretory process; if you use super-strong antiperspirants under the arms, you may find you develop back acne and chest acne and even spots on the lower jaw, because the body has to get rid of those toxins somehow.

- Dial down to a normal deodorant, rather than an antiperspirant; try roll-ons with essential oils, found in natural food stores. This is an adjustment that takes time, but the sweat glands *will* rebalance.

- Add a few drops of tea tree oil to the body wash you use under your arms (or buy a tea tree-based wash), and use on a daily basis. Leave it under your arms while you wash hair etc so it has time to work. Soap and water alone don't have adequate antibacterial agents so although they'll remove the surface sweat, they're not neutralising the bacteria; you'll feel clean for half an hour and then the smell boomerangs back.

- If you want a quick boost while out and about, you can put 3–4 drops of tea tree onto your palms and rub into the underarm area (it is one of the few essential oils that can be used neat on skin).

- Some fabrics are much better than others for managing sweat. Cotton and other natural fabrics breathe and absorb sweat, allowing it to dry quickly. Choose bamboo or cotton in your workout clothes instead. Many synthetics don't breathe as well (ironically since many athletic clothes are made of synthetics), although the leading sportswear and athletic-wear companies now do offer breathable fabrics that 'wick away' sweat, and it's worth paying the extra.

- If you know you're going to be in a nervous situation, or are not sure what the temperature of the room will be, layer your clothes, such as with a jacket that can be taken off, to save any embarrassment.

And remember: it's normal to sweat!

Cellulite

Cellulite refers to fat and fluid that's collected in specific areas to give a bumpy, lumpy look. It mostly builds up on hips, thighs and buttocks, with perhaps a little on the tummy or the top of the arms.

When we retain fluid (perhaps through weight gain), the number of fat and fluid cells doesn't change, so fluid gets trapped between the cells and that's what gives the dimpling. The first step is to do more topical work on the areas with cellulite, with body brushing, body scrub and body lotion, to see if that brings about improvements. Get everything moving in the area! If that doesn't do the trick, though, we need to add more ingredients and extra techniques:

- Certain ingredients are famous for their impact on cellulite: ivy, butcher's broom and caffeine as well as essential oils (lemongrass, juniper, fennel, grapefruit). Look for them on ingredients lists of the oils and creams you'll be applying, or the scrubs you'll use to massage the area. Essential oil-based cellulite products actually make you wee more often, so don't use these in the morning before your commute to work!

- The other effective action is to increase circulation in the area, because typically, cellulite happens in areas of sluggish circulation. Body brush daily (see p.257 for technique). There are also machines and in-salon treatments such as endermologie, high-energy radial shockwave and laser treatments, as well as courses of targeted physical massage treatments, if nothing else is working, but they're a big investment in terms of both time and money.

- Using self-tanner will also help to disguise the appearance of cellulite, but you need to do the whole body, or all of the legs/arms, not only the affected areas, of course, so the results appear seamless.

I want to reassure you: nobody thinks your cellulite is as bad as you do. We're so self-critical, yet other people are looking at the whole picture, probably admiring your swimming costume, rather than thinking: 'Look at that dimpling!' Certainly, don't ever let it make you so self-conscious that it stops you enjoying life and getting in that pool.

Sensitive body skin

If skin seems infected and inflamed, is very itchy and cracked, you should consult your doctor; it may be a medical condition they can sort out with a prescription.

If you usually have comfortable skin, you can experience sensitive skin and flare-ups on the body just as easily as you can on the face area. The best thing is to work backwards and figure out what might have caused it:

- Is it where clothing is quite tight or rubs, like a bra strap, around waistbands or elbow/knee creases?

- Could it be the fabric of the clothing itself? I always recommend wearing natural fabrics, rather than synthetics.

- Is it the washing powder or fabric conditioner you've been using, especially if you've switched lately? Sometimes we can have a reaction to laundry products used when we've stayed in a hotel or a friend's house.

I'm afraid you do need to become a bit of a detective, here, to try to figure out what the trigger is. (See my 'trigger list', p.99.)

Here are some things that can help to calm your skin:

- Use calming, soothing, desensitising ingredients like calamine, aloe vera, lavender, allantoin or calendula, which now come in easy-to-use, quick-drying gels and oils. Also use 'clean' and 'free-from' formulas.

- If sensitivity is sweat-related, use antiseptic washes on those areas, dry thoroughly and keep the area dry with a cornstarch-based powder, but make sure the area is absolutely bone dry before applying, otherwise you're creating the perfect environment for bacteria and fungi to breed.

- Dial up exfoliation to take away the dead skin cells, then apply a rich moisturising oil or butter. Shea butter and oils like jojoba, argan and vitamin E can work wonders.

- If your skin is irritated in areas where you're removing hair, e.g. bikini line, leg area, underarm or the back, take a look at your hair removal method. Use antiseptic wipes before hair removal; don't apply perfume, aftershave, deodorant or any other scented product before or after hair removal; and look at different ways that could work for you without causing rash and irritation.

Spotty bodies

Spots can affect many different areas of the body, not just your face. You can suffer from acne as an adult (see p.108), but your spots may be due to other reasons, so I suggest going into detective mode, and if they're worrying you seek medical advice.

- Are they painless, dry, raised and perhaps red, but there's nothing to come out if you were to try to squeeze them? This may not be acne, but instead *Keratosis pilaris* (see Ask Alison, p.280).

- Are the spots on the thighs, legs and sometimes the chest? Well, these kind of spots tend to be a symptom of dry skin build-up. The test is to exfoliate the affected area/s three nights in a row, then smooth in as rich a moisturiser or body moisturiser as you own. You'll see an improvement as early as the first day, but definitely by day three, in which case your body's telling you that you need to be putting on moisturiser on a daily basis. Try moisturisers with built-in exfoliators, such as AHAs (see p.115).

- If the spots are sore, infected and raised, and if you were to squeeze them, something would come out, then that is a form of acne on the body. Try using the same products as you do on your face for blackheads and breakouts, or try blue light treatments.

- If the spots are in the form of small red pimples – more like a rash than breakouts – add an antiseptic wash into your body regime. Be sure to wash the flannel each time you use it. That may be all it takes to improve the look and manage the problem.

Beautiful hands

Hands work hard. They're in and out of water, exposed to UV light, soap and paper towels (which sap any moisture), garden soil, paint etc. and nowadays, lashings of sanitiser. Happily, even the driest, most lacklustre hands can be transformed with just a little TLC. So here's how…

Did you know that the skin on your hands is thinner than the skin on your face? It's more like the thickness of an eyelid, actually, so it's no wonder hands can age faster than the face. (They do say that a glance at your hands is a bigger age giveaway than a sneaky peek at the date of birth in our passport!)

Here are the daily handcare 'musts'…

Cuticle care

Oiling your nails and cuticles is fantastic for nail health and strength. The massage action brings blood to the nail, will deliver a wonderful shine even if you're not a nail-painter, and you'll never need your cuticles clipped if you're oiling and massaging them regularly. I've found that the more cuticles are clipped, the more they grow back, so I'm not a fan, even though I'm a qualified nail technician. Discourage manicurists who are eager to cut cuticles, especially if you're having nails done as a one-off, say, for a holiday or big event, because the cuticles will grow back thicker and more obvious than before. It's fine if you're prepared to have regular manicures, because these will deal with cuticle regrowth, but otherwise, avoid.

Cleaning up the cuticle area creates a much more groomed 'frame' for varnish. If you haven't really paid attention to your cuticles till now and they're thick and dry, there are some brilliant cuticle dissolvers out there; pop them on for 30 seconds or so and push the cuticles back with a round-ended rubber hoof stick, which will remove any excess skin and debris.

Filing

Still using the old emery board style of nail file? You'll find a crystal file life-changing. Reach for it whenever you feel a nick or a catch in your nails, as well as during a manicure itself. Keep it in its protective sleeve, because this type of file can snap easily, if you're not careful. There are so many variables with traditional nail files in terms of the level of sand and grit, whereas a crystal file is 100 per cent fool-proof.

A regular nail file should never be used in a see-sawing motion because this can lift the layers of the nail and damage them, causing a little 'earthquake' in the nail which can result in breaks further down, below the tip of the nail. But with a crystal file, a see-sawing action's fine for smoothing, and much easier to use if you're not a trained technician.

The most flattering look for nails is a shape that mirrors the look of your nail bed. If you have a long, oval nail bed, you can get away with longer, oval nails, if you choose. If the base of your nails is square, you'll look better with square, softly-rounded edges. Don't try to file nails from long to short; use a nail clipper first to reduce length. Use a really small clipper for your hands, not a toenail clipper which will completely invert the nail when you press down, cracking and splitting it. Make small clipping movements around the nail, then file afterwards to smooth out the rough edges.

Protect with SPF

Spending any time outside? Whatever facial SPF you're using, put it on the backs of your hands (and the tops of your feet). Hands are more prone to age spots than the face itself, and you want to take SPF out with you for reapplying because (unlike the face), you're washing hands several times a day. Some hand creams have SPF too.

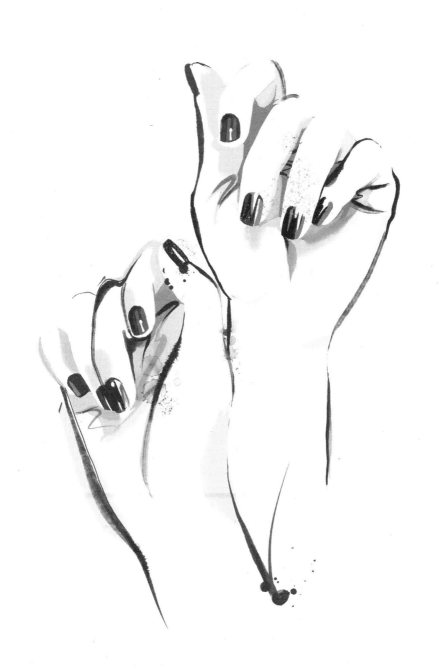

Nourish and moisturise

Hands will lap up any excess face product you are using, whether a mask, moisturiser or scrub, so don't miss them out! They work so hard for you; reward them! Ideally, you want to own lots of hand creams, because you want them handy (!). I have hand cream on my desk, in the car, next to the remote control, by washbasins (I prefer pump creams next to taps, for ease). Most important of all is the hand cream on your bedside table, for a generous pre-sleep massage that allows a really thick, generous layer of cream to sink in overnight.

When you apply hand cream, don't just squirt it into the palms of your hands and rub together. Instead, apply it to the *back* of your hands and rub the backs together to distribute. Then use your fingers to massage the cream into your fingers and nails, and take 30 seconds to push the cream into the cuticles, gently easing them back. Palms have their own secretions so only need a little moisturising, so use the very last residue of your hand cream on your palms.

Hand sanitiser

We have got into the good habit of using hand sanitiser, whether at school, work, in shops, restaurants etc. When buying sanitiser, look for one with the World Health Organisation recommended alcohol level of 60 per cent minimum for a protective action against germs, and ideally find a brand that includes moisturising ingredients like glycerine or aloe vera to counter any drying action. Many find hand sanitisers can cause instant dryness and soreness. If this happens to you, do a full hand treatment nightly. If your skin seems to cope fine, still moisturise; like sun damage, ageing and pigmentation can emerge years later.

Alison's Tip ————————————————————

I'm not a fan of rubber gloves, which I feel make hands hot and sweaty, especially if you're eczema- or sensitive-skin-prone, like me. Instead, look for natural cleaning products and switch to those, because they'll almost certainly be kinder to hands. You can put back any lost moisture afterwards with hand cream. Gloves, for me, are for when you really need protection, for example, when gardening, to stop soil from getting under nails and to shield against cuts and grazes. I definitely wear gloves when I'm riding my horses, to avoid calluses.

DIY manicure

You can achieve an almost salon-perfect manicure at home. It might take a little practice, but here's your step-by-step…

Take your time. Don't even think of giving yourself a manicure if you're going to have to cook dinner or drive somewhere soon; an at-home manicure is best done after an early supper and a few hours before bedtime, to allow nails to dry properly.

1 **Shape your nails.** I don't use polish remover before shaping my nails; instead, I leave the polish on until after I've shaped them. This is for two reasons: firstly, because they're stronger, and secondly, it makes it easier to judge the right shape and to match them. If you have bare nails, it's good to shape them before soaking, as otherwise the layers are more prone to peeling. After shaping, remove polish, if you have it on. See p.267 for shaping tips.

2 **Soften rough skin.** Soak your hands in a basin of warm water for several minutes (or take a shower at this point). I like to add milk or milk powder because the lactic acid in the milk helps dissolve dead cells and softens cuticles, while the natural fats are also good for dry skin.

3   **Push back your cuticles.** Apply cuticle remover; then, using a hoof stick or an angle-tipped nail stick lightly wrapped in a whisper of cotton wool, gently push your cuticles back towards the base of the nail. There is no need to clip them (see p.266).

4   **Buff your nails until they gleam.** Buffing nails creates a wonderfully smooth, glassy surface that gives a shinier effect when you polish. Look for one of the multi-surface buffers which has numbers on it, indicating which order to use the different areas of the buffer in, from roughest to finest. Gently buff the whole nail, using a side-to-side motion and don't allow heat to build up.

5   **Clean nails.** If you're going to be using nail polish, you need a grease-free surface for the polish to adhere to. I like to scrub nails at this point with a nail brush, soap and water.

6   **Apply strengthener/base coat.** Apply nail strengthener if you have flaky, weak nails. Then apply a base coat (or use a combination product with base coat included).

NOTE: Some brands offer all-in-one products which are base coat, colour and top coat in one, for time-saving.

7   **Apply one or two coats of polish.** Some top brands now give great results with a single coat, but whichever you choose, work from bottom to top. Try to apply each coat in just two to three strokes.

8   **Apply top coat.** Take this over the top tip of the nail, all the way underneath the free edge, to seal the tip and add longevity to your manicure. The best way to ensure a manicure lasts is to reapply top coat every two or three days, to keep your nails shiny and to protect both the colour and the nail itself.

LOOKING AFTER YOUR POLISHES

You have bought a gorgeous nail polish colour. Here are my 'musts' for keeping it looking its best:

- Clean the neck of the bottle each time before you use it, with polish remover, to remove any semi-dried bits.

- Rather than shake the bottle, roll it between your hands to agitate and ensure it's perfectly mixed.

- Always keep your polishes upright rather than in a jumble in a drawer or bag.

- I am not a fan of keeping polish in the fridge; I have nail varnishes I've had for six or seven years without them going blobby, and they really will last for ages if you just keep them out of direct sunlight, upright and away from heat.

- If you find a particular shape of brush that you like, save the brush when you've finished the polish. Give it a deep clean in polish remover poured into the cap of the bottle, and use it with your other brands of polish. You can also buy different shaped nail application brushes from nail websites.

9   **Apply quick-dry.** Wait a couple of minutes after the top
    coat and drop a single drop of cuticle oil onto each nail and
    super-lightly spread it over the nail surface. If your cuticle oil
    has a brush, you can use it to paint the oil over the surface.
    You can actually do this with any oil, to turbo-charge drying
    time; it also stops fluff from sticking to your manicure.

10 **Moisturise and massage.** I like to wait for nails to be
    completely dry before working a favourite cream or a base
    oil like sweet almond oil, avocado or olive oil into my hands.

11 **Avoid soaking afterwards in hot water.** Don't have a bath
    after a manicure or pedicure. Nail varnish is designed to dry
    quickly, but the underlying layers take a few hours to dry
    and if you expose them to hot water, the layers will lift more
    readily and you'll shorten the lifespan of your hard work.

AGE-DEFYING POLISH

A glossy nail is a young-looking nail. That shine might be from buffing,
or a glossy polish shade from nude to dark. Ridged, discoloured nails do
not look great. Shade-wise, I think that women (and men) of any age look
great in high-fashion colours, because it shows you've got your finger
(literally) on the pulse of what's stylish. If you're not brave enough to do
that on your fingers, then toes look great in bold and dazzling shades.
Every season now has a teal, an orange, a plum... Experiment! But also
find 'your' perfect nude shade that enhances your skin tone. Take your
cue from your favourite nude lipstick and find something similar for nails.

Alison's Tip

If you snap a nail or have to cut it down because of damage, take down the length of all your nails with clippers, then file to even them up. Having one or two short nails when the others are long just draws attention to the fact you've broken one.

Putting your best foot forwards

Happy feet really do make for a happier person, yet feet are so often neglected and forgotten. Over a lifetime, they'll carry you hundreds of thousands of miles. You can ensure they feel comfortable and look really attractive, with just a few simple steps.

Exfoliate, exfoliate, exfoliate

What makes feet happiest, if you ask me? Removing the hard skin that builds up when we walk, jog, run, exercise or wear shoes that put pressure on particular places on the feet.

Some people just aren't hard skin 'producers' and may never need to buff their feet to keep them comfortable. But if you do have hard skin, check out the brilliant battery-powered foot files, which whizz over the foot causing almost a snowdrift of dead skin to come off. Alternatively, you can manually remove hard skin with a metal foot file, but be sure it's not too 'grater-like', because the rougher the file, the more skin it will remove (you don't want to take off too much skin and leave your feet sore). The skin that comes off should be fine as dust – and you may want to protect your floor from it with a towel, by the way.

If you've got hard skin that has taken weeks, months or even years to build up, don't try to remove it all at once; it's better to take it off in twice-weekly sessions, over a few weeks. You could also consider a foot peel mask or exfoliating sock: these feature combinations of acids which soften and dissolve the layers, and when you remove them, the top layers of skin just roll off. (I sometimes take these on holiday with me to get my feet beach-ready if I haven't had time for a pedicure beforehand. They're a good fast fix.)

Last thing at night, give yourself a foot massage

As a reflexologist, I can access the health of the whole body through the soles of the feet. I know just how important self-care of the feet is, and how much difference a nightly foot rub can make to overall wellbeing. It's easy to think: 'I'm too tired for this…' – but I promise you, you'll get a better night's sleep if you take just a few minutes to rub cream into your feet last thing. You can buy a specific foot cream, or use anything you've got that's rich and buttery, perhaps with cocoa or shea butters.

Soaking your feet

I am a big fan of soaking your feet each night, especially if you are on your feet all day. Where have all the electric foot spas gone, I wonder? They were brilliant for this. However, a good old washing-up bowl is the next best thing. Soak for 10 minutes in warm-to-hot water (not uncomfortably hot), infused with magnesium salts (available in big, economical bags) or an arnica soak. You could also use soothing essential oils like peppermint, basil, ginger and geranium, which are just so good for achiness and tiredness. Tea tree is great if you have smelly feet.

A foot bath soothes the nerve ends of the body and takes away the pressure; shoes are a sort of bondage, really. If you're a shower person rather than a bath-lover, you'll really benefit from a good foot soak at night, especially if you're standing on a hard, concrete floor all day, such as in retail or as a medical professional.

Between pedicures, brush around the cuticles daily with an old toothbrush if you're in the bath or shower. Sounds weird, but this is softer than a nail brush and helps to get rid of dead skin – it's amazing what a difference you'll see in just a week.

Look out for infections

'Winter' shoes and boots – not to mention trainers – don't allow for air circulation. And because feet sweat, they create the perfect environment for fungal infections like athlete's foot. Trainers and wellies are the worst culprit because they're made of synthetic materials and are sealed in and hot, like mini-saunas. Make sure after you wash your feet that they are thoroughly dry, perhaps dusting on cornstarch-based powder or an antiseptic foot powder. Change your socks every day, and allow shoes 24 hours to dry out between wears; even when you think they're dry, they're really not. Avoid going barefoot in areas where infections lurk, like in changing rooms or around pools – flip-flops are always a safer choice. Antiseptic foot lotions are also helpful – and you might not immediately think of it, but hand sanitisers are also foot sanitisers! So spritz generously, and massage in. If you do get a foot infection, your first step is your local pharmacy where you should be able to find specialist podiatry products; some also have resident podiatrists who they may refer you to.

DIY pedicure

A salon pedicure at the start of summer kicks off the sandal season beautifully. But if you haven't the time or budget, you can give yourself happy, shiny toes...

1 **First, shape your nails.** Toenails should be clipped straight across, but don't try and clip the whole nail in one go with a large clipper. Use short snips. Even up the shape with a nail file.

2 **Remove old polish.** Remove all polish using acetone-free nail polish remover and cotton wool pads. If you're wearing shimmer or glitter polish, press the soaked cotton pad down on the nails for several seconds to flood the toenail, before trying to remove the polish. Little flecks of glitter, which can be left behind even after you're removed a glitter polish, can be almost 'flicked' off the nail with the tip of a crystal nail file.

3 **Remove hard skin.** Lay a towel on the floor under your feet to catch the dead skin you're dislodging. Use your foot file (battery-operated or hand-held, see p.274) and work on areas of hard skin.

4 **Soak your feet.** Soak your feet in warm water (see p.275). Add a specialist foot soak, a handful of milk powder (or some fresh milk), or some magnesium salts, and/or a few drops of essential oils – peppermint is good if feet are tired. Swish and soak your feet for up to 10 minutes.

5 **Sort out your cuticles.** Apply cuticle remover and push back your cuticles gently (see manicure, p.270). Apply cuticle oil. If you don't have a specific cuticle oil, a base oil like argan or apricot kernel does the trick.

6 **Moisturise, moisturise, moisturise.** Feet have no oil glands, so they drink moisture and respond beautifully to rich textures like shea butter and coconut oil. More is more is more.

7 **Apply polish.** Wipe each nail first to remove oil. See DIY manicure for these steps, through to finishing with a quick-dry spray or a nail oil (see p.270). You can choose clear or colours – whatever you like!

Hey, presto! Your feet can be transformed in a few blinks of an eye – and there's something so cheering about looking down at prettier toes.

There's something so cheering about looking down at prettier toes.

Ask Alison: body matters Q&A

Have I ever been stopped in a supermarket and asked about 'chicken skin'? You bet – and they weren't asking about something in their shopping trolley. So here's what I answer, to that and other pressing body beauty queries…

Q: How do I 'layer' body products?

It's an echo of the ritual for the face: thin to thick. A serum or gel goes on first, followed by an oil, followed by cream, lotion or butter. If you want to use a firming, anti-cellulite product and a 'designer' fragranced body lotion, say, the treatment product would go on first, always.

Q: I've got an operation scheduled. How can I prepare my skin?

First and foremost, of course, follow your doctor's advice. But basically, you want to get the skin into the most moisturised, supple, soft condition that you possibly can because if you do, you won't scar so much afterwards. That means regular exfoliation and upping your body moisturising regime so you're layering on an oil with a cream or butter on top, and ideally reapplying several times a day, if you're at home. If you're out and about, it's more challenging – but you can decant a cream/butter into a small, portable container and pop it in your bag or man bag. Alternatively, you can break open a capsule of vitamin E and smooth into the area that's going to be operated on; capsules, of course, are ideal for carrying around with you. And absolutely no sunbathing on a pre-op area as it will dry it out.

Q: What's your advice for healing scars?

Once the stitches are out and you've got the go-ahead from your doctor to start applying products of your own, slather on vitamin E moisturising gels and creams. Twice a day really isn't enough. It's really important to gently massage a scar; it helps to prevent it thickening, particularly relevant if you want to avoid keloid (raised) scarring. Scars heal for months after an operation; in fact, the healing is still going on for at least a year afterwards because the cells have been traumatised in the most brutal way, deep down. During that time you must absolutely avoid exposing it to the sun, because a scar can coarsen, thicken or darken, as a result. I often hear people say, 'I'll just get some sun on it; that'll help' – but the opposite is true. Cover your scar with an SPF50+ and if you can't cover it up with clothing, put a hankie or a scarf over it to shield it. A scar needs to heal for at least a year before you expose it to sun.

Q: What can I do to prevent ingrown hairs?

Ingrown hairs happen when a hair is blocked by dead skin cells on the surface, and turns back on itself and grows back into the body in a sort of curl, instead. Increase exfoliation in areas that are prone to ingrown hairs such as legs and bikini line; you can do this with an exfoliating scrub, or liquid peel pads. That will prevent the cells building up on the surface so hairs don't get trapped.

Q: My breasts are sagging, what can I do?

What a lot of people don't realise is that breast tissue has no muscle of its own; your breasts are made up of one-third mammary cells and two-thirds fat, held together by fascia and a skin 'envelope', and supported by muscle underneath. So any movement of the bust area steadily stretches the skin. You don't have to have a large bust to have a slack bust; it's all about the movement, which stretches the skin and tissues.

Chest exercises are good for firming the muscles above the bust, which can change the shape of the area above your breasts, but don't expect them to have any impact on firmness or pertness of the breasts themselves. However, you can definitely see a difference with bust firming products and you can even measure the improvements, if you need convincing. Look into a mirror and push one breast up as far as it will go. Draw on your sternum with a dot of eyeliner pencil, in line with your nipple. Then push your breast downwards, as far as it will go, and mark the nipple-line there, on the sternum. If you have what is considered a firm bust, you'll see anything from 1–5cm movement, but I've seen people with 13cm movement. It's not related to breast size because you can have small, slack breasts or larger, firmer breasts. It's down to skin quality and how much everything's been stretched (often by breastfeeding). Try this measuring again a few weeks after using the firming products, to see progress.

You can invest in specific breast-firming products, or use a regular body firming product (if you want to maintain the size of your bust) or a cellulite treatment (if you want to take the size down – the breasts can be affected by fluid retention, too). You've got to put in the time: these products don't work by magic, and require twice-daily application if you want to see an uplift.

Be sure that your bra fits really well, to stop any movement pulling on the underlying supportive muscles – and if you do any kind of vigorous exercise, wear a sports bra, without fail, or swap to something low-impact like swimming. Wearing a high SPF on your chest, just like your face, is also key, as sun damage slackens the skin that supports the bust.

It's now accepted that we come in all sorts of different shapes and sizes, so don't get hung up about not having the 'perfect' breasts, and try to avoid comparing yourself with others, always. Mostly, so-called 'perfect' breasts have cost their owner thousands of pounds in cosmetic surgery! But in real life, boobs and eyebrows are very individual, rarely match perfectly – and anyone who criticises yours isn't worth knowing.

Q: I have 'chicken skin' – what can I do about it?

Keratosis pilaris is the official name for areas of rough, dehydrated, almost little 'mountain peaks' of skin. It tends to show up in areas of bulky muscle, like upper arms, thighs and the bum, where the bulk of the muscle can affect circulation. Sometimes it's just dehydrated skin, rather than actual KP, and there is a lot you can do at home. Dial up the exfoliation to at least twice a week and moisturise daily. Take any of your AHA body lotions (glycolic can be particularly effective), or even facial products like peel pads or liquid facial peels if you have them, and wipe over the area. Combined with improved moisturising, this can be very effective at reducing the 'chicken skin' appearance, but if the problem's still there after a month, check in with your doctor.

Q: What can I do about a wrinkled neck/décolletage?

This is a huge area of concern for so many because the chest area is just so perfectly angled to the sun to pick up sun damage, which can result in crêpiness, sagging and even a sort of 'paving slab' wrinkling.

My first rule is to double up: take your neck products down at least as far as the 'scoop-neck-t-shirt' line, and take all body products up to the jawline. Almost every leading skincare range now offers a targeted neck treatment, but the amounts prescribed are for average maintenance rather than for playing catch-up. So: apply more than the pot says, and apply it more often, probably more than twice a day. Layer on an SPF50+ on the whole area each and every morning to help prevent future damage.

For a bigger investment, there are also targeted Intense Pulsed Light machines or lasers for home use. Leaving aside the financial investment, you also realistically have to be prepared to invest the time in using them.

If you're going out, you can plump up the area with a rich moisturiser or neck cream just before getting dressed to improve its appearance. You could even give your neck a mini neck-and-décolletage facial, with a mask, serum and a moisturiser, which will make it look a hundred times better, short-term. Then use a matte bronzer to match up face, neck and chest, or a foundation or body make-up that doesn't come off on clothes.

Q: What's the advice for rough elbows?

Elbows are a friction area, rubbing against clothing, being rested on tables… Illness can also cause rough elbows. On different skin tones, the skin may appear darker or lighter. It sounds obvious, but moisturiser really helps; every time you're applying to your face or hands, try to remember to lavish some product on your elbows.

Whenever you squeeze a lemon for a recipe, you can use the two halves for a fruit acid treatment; literally rest your elbows in the lemon hulls – a free peel! Exfoliating peel pads with AHAs, most notably glycolic, can also be effective.

Q: How can I rehab my nails after shellac or acrylics?

Some nails actually benefit from the reinforcement of shellac or acrylics and grow stronger, but others can take two to three months to recover. You will have been used to having a strongly reinforced nail, but the natural nails below can be soft – you may well also have had several layers buffed off by your nail technician, and it's the buffing work that can be damaging. So ask them to be gentle, and never get the shellac/acrylics buffed off – you want them dissolved. To get your nails back into tip-top condition, nourishing nail oils, nail strengtheners and cuticle removers are your best friends. You may also want to take a nail supplement, to strengthen from within.

Q: Any tips to prepare for hair removal?

If you're going for waxing, exfoliate the area two or three times a week, beforehand (although not on the day), and moisturise afterwards to ensure the skin is supple. Patch testing is a must. If you're using a product at home for the first time, be sure to patch test. If you're going to a salon, you'll need to pop in beforehand for the test, or the salon may be able to organise a home patch test to be sent out. Better safe than sorry.

Q: How do I use body make-up?

Body make-up can be great for boosting confidence; for covering up scars, thread veins, improving the appearance of varicose veins, as well as evening out skin tone in such a smooth way that it looks completely natural. I promise you I have the worst corned beef legs with varicose veining and if they come out, it's only thanks to body make-up.

There have been such huge improvements in body make-up in the past few years, so if you had a bad experience in the past, it's definitely time to try again. Nowadays, formulations look much more realistic, often available in a range of skin tone-matched shades. Because they're waterproof, they literally don't budge for days, or until you scrub with soap and water, unlike the earlier versions that came off on your clothes immediately. It's worth researching the brands they use on film sets.

You also have products in your make-up kit that can double up on the body: bronzers, in the form of powders or creams or gels, or highlighters. A little bit of highlighter or shimmer looks fantastic smoothed lightly onto skin to draw attention to shoulders, forearms or décolletage – whichever areas you're happy with and want to draw attention to. A particularly good trick is a tiny bit of highlighter down the front of the shins to lengthen the look of the leg.

Q: My hands/feet are super dry. What should I do?

Dry hands are especially common after a lot of hand washing and sanitising, gardening, DIY or illness. Here is my intense catch-up treatment for super dry skin – make sure you have a bit of time and everything to hand before you start!

- Exfoliate the hands or feet with a granular exfoliant, or sugar mixed in olive oil.
- Rinse and apply coconut or olive oil, then a thick layer of moisturiser.
- Wrap your hands/feet in cling film or two polythene bags, and put a pair of socks on over the top to keep it all in place.
- Hold your hands/feet over the top of a hot water bottle while you leave the moisturiser to sink in for 15 minutes, or longer if you wish.
- Remove the socks and cling film/bags, and massage in any residue left on the skin. If you're immediately painting your nails, remove any oil/moisturiser from the nails first with nail varnish remover.

The golden rules

"

The sun needs to be treated with a healthy respect

The sun is a life force. But, wonderful as it makes us feel, it needs to be treated with respect. Whether you like to tan naturally or prefer a faux glow, here's what you need to know...

Sunlight is good for us. It has a massive anti-depressive effect. It gives us natural vitamin D, known to be vital for our immune systems. And that warmth makes people feel so g-o-o-d. All of which means that the sun isn't something to be frightened of, but it does, nevertheless, need to be treated with a healthy respect. Short, sharp bursts of exposure still traumatise the skin, triggering swelling, redness and ultimately, sunburn and sun damage.

Because of its famous feel-good factor, I know many people who love to bask in sunshine. I've never really been able to do that because strong sunlight can give me a migraine. Oh, I tried to tan, when I was younger, but since I spent most of my life in jodhpurs, I never did get those golden-brown legs. Besides, I lived in the North of England, wind whipping off the sea, where anoraks are considered summer wear. At the time, a deep, dark tan was very fashionable. That 'old-fashioned' tan generally traumatised the skin, which went red and peeled. Happily, nowadays, there's less pressure to do that because every skin tone under the sun is now represented in advertising, including porcelain pale. Anything goes and there is no real 'pressure' or fashion to tan nowadays.

No question: over-exposure to UV light is linked with lines, wrinkles, age spots and slackening. It takes 10 years for most of that UV damage to appear, so you may think you've got away scot-free, while in reality, the effects of that exposure are just biding their time.

I am so often asked by young twenty-somethings: 'What's the best anti-ageing product for my skin?' I always answer: 'An SPF30 day cream, ideally a higher SPF than that. Every day. And SPF50 on holiday, for sure.'

Don't be that person standing in the queue for your flight back with a flaking, red, peeling and angry tan. In my book, an 'expensive-looking' tan is when your skin is a skin-kissed shade but is in great, glowing condition.

Whether you want to achieve a gradual natural glow, or fake it with one of the self-tanning products on the market, is entirely up to you. But what I can say is that the products to help you achieve your 'perfect' tan have never been better, easier to use, or have delivered such good results, as now.

The natural tan

The safest tan of all is a fake tan. But because of sun's feel-good factor, many of us want to expose our skin to the rays of the sun itself. The key to a tan that lasts – and is as safe as possible – is to do so slowly, patiently and with the right protective products. You can even get a deeper tan this way. Here's how…

Use a tan accelerator

Tan accelerator is an innovation that has made a splash in the last few years. These products are a hit because they really work. They stimulate melanin production in your skin so that when you do get out in the sun, the pigment is ready both as protection, and to darken more quickly. You're basically enhancing your body's own protection so that if you're someone who burns on day one, even with sun protection, that's less likely to happen (though of course you still need your normal SPF applied in the usual way). You'll also tan more evenly if you're someone who tends to pick up a patchy tan. And if you suffer from urticaria (prickly heat), as I have, I find these can also be a godsend.

My advice is to start using a tan accelerator body lotion in the spring, and use it through until autumn. If not, do at least use one in the run-up to your summer holiday for two weeks. And if you don't want your tan to fade continue to use them after your holiday and at the end of summer, too. Try to get one that can also act as an aftersun and has the right level of moisturiser for your skin, so you can use it as your body lotion for a while.

Use more SPF than you think you need

The general advice is at least a shot glass-full for the body for each application – roughly equivalent to a generously heaped dessertspoonful, if you're not a tequila drinker! When testing SPFs, labs apply way more thickly than we do in normal life, so we need to be very generous. For faces, apply much more lavishly than you would a normal moisturiser. If you wish, you can buy an SPF formula with tan accelerator in it, or even a tint/shimmer – there's so much choice.

Apply your SPF before breakfast

Getting from hotel or apartment to the beach or pool can take time, as can finding your spot when you get there, and suddenly, you realise you've been out in the sun, exposed, for an hour without realising. So whatever type of protection you choose, apply it before you even step outside in the morning. Also ensure it's in your flight bag as, again, that sunburn can begin when you land if there are long transfers or delays.

I prefer a once-a-day SPF formula

If you haven't tried one, let me tell you: they can be pretty darned transformational for you and your family. Once-a-days can also prevent arguments with kids, who generally hate having sun care applied and it's hard to pull them away from beach and pool activities to reapply protection several times a day. Once-a-days are also good for sending kids off to school protected in the morning. Excellent for people who work outdoors, too – for instance in construction – as well as anyone who's involved in sports.

The golden rule: sun care must be applied to cool, non-sweaty skin in order to 'seal' the formula on the skin. Wait at least half an hour after showering to apply a once-a-day, because the skin continues to sweat for that time. You really need to be in a dry environment for them to 'bond' to skin, too, so if you're staying somewhere humid and you don't have air conditioning, a once-a-day may not be right for you. Once sealed, though, they won't come off in water and they will survive a natural air-drying after swimming, although be aware, no sunscreen survives vigorous towel-rubbing, so you will need to reapply.

Sunscreens work best on exfoliated skin, so get the whole family using an exfoliator twice a week before your holiday. Otherwise you'll be sealing the SPF to dead skin cells, which can rub off more easily and drastically affect the protective effects. Also avoid spraying perfume or deodorant over the protected skin as these can stop the SPF from working and cause sun sensitivity and pigmentation.

Avoid the hours between 11am and 3pm

That's when you're most likely to burn. I know it's tempting: your holiday's short. Head off and have your lunch under the shade of a tree or a parasol; one of the great joys of a holiday, if you ask me. Or go sightseeing, wearing a hat and loose cover-up clothing.

Trust me: you will still tan in the shade

Sun reflects off sand, water or the tiles round a pool, right onto your skin. A shade-acquired tan is the safest tan of all, because you're at less risk of burning. I can put my hand on my heart and promise you that you *will* develop a beautiful, lasting tan over the duration of your holiday, even out of direct sun.

Alison's Tip

Place a towel on your sun lounger. This not only absorbs sweat, but also avoids picking up fungal infections from the synthetic surface of the lounger. As an extra safeguard, first spritz your lounger with your hand sanitiser.

If you're using a regular sunscreen, top it up often

The protective ingredients in regular sunscreens (rather than once-a-day types) start to degrade almost as soon as you put them on. So you should really reapply every 30–40 minutes, before going in the water, and again when you've towel-dried. If you're swimming in a chlorinated pool, then shower before reapplying sunscreen.

Buy sunscreen before you travel.

You'll be able to buy products from ranges you know, like and trust, rather than being faced with a sea of unfamiliar products with foreign instructions in an international pharmacy or supermarket.

Be aware of extra-vulnerable bits

These are areas of thin or no hair coverage (a bald head, a wide parting, back of neck); ears; hands; tops of feet; tops of knees, chest – all are perfectly angled to pick up sun damage. The chest is so vulnerable that when brands test anti-ageing products, they often do it on the décolletage because it generally ages so much more than the face. Be even more generous with sun care applications on all of these areas, using the same SPF as the face.

The slower a tan develops, the longer it will last

If you try to speed things up, you'll burn, then peel. So take it easy at the start of a holiday.

Stick with the same SPF throughout your holiday

Simplify your life and your tanning by taking one level of SPF and sticking to it from start to finish. Ideally, I'd recommend an SPF50+, or at the very least, SPF30; SPF20 certainly isn't adequate (especially for the face). Once again, you have to trust me that you will still tan with a higher number. It'll happen more slowly, but it will last longer and you'll inflict less damage on your skin. Try it next time you're away and I promise you'll see I'm right. (SPFs are now available with built-in tan accelerator, which will speed things up.)

When you're reapplying SPF, swipe away the previous layer with a facial wipe or cotton pads soaked in micellar water that you keep in a little plastic container (like a lunchbox), otherwise you'll trap sweat and grime between the layers, which may trigger outbreaks.

Take shade breaks

If you absolutely can't resist lying out in the sun, add in shade breaks to allow skin to cool down. It really does help to avoid a sunburn.

Certain products don't mix with sunshine

Avoid wearing perfume, perfumed body products, antiperspirants or deodorants when sunbathing; the chemicals can interact with UV light. Also avoid retinols, glycolics or peels, which leave skin more vulnerable. On a sun holiday, use your serum and moisturising treatments at night-time. Strong-coloured lipsticks are also a bad idea because the heat can melt the formula, which will travel beyond the lips.

Be generous with the aftersun

When you get back to your room, shower to remove any chlorine, grime or salt from skin (and hair). Pat skin until it's dry or just damp before applying aftersun. Then apply lavish amounts of aftersun – an absolute skin-saver.

ESSENTIAL BEACH KIT

Here's a checklist for packing your favourite beach basket or tote:

- A large sunhat.
- Baseball cap for sports.
- Sunglasses – ideally large, dark sunglasses with wide arms, which can help shield the vulnerable eye area from sun damage.
- Hammam towels – these lightweight towels dry quickly, but are also useful for draping over a sun lounger or lightly over the body, if you want to protect it. Big, fluffy towels are fine for the hotel room, but heavy to lug to the beach.
- Sunscreen for face and for body.
- Toner or micellar cleanser with cotton pads (for cleansing skin between facial reapplications).
- Large bottle of water, to stay hydrated.
- Kimono or other cover-up.
- SPF lip balm.

If you're on a hiking holiday, skiing or city break, remember to pack the sunscreen, sunglasses, SPF lip balm, plenty of water to stay hydrated, and in hot weather, a hat that shields your face.

Many aftersun products boast calming, soothing, heat-dispersing ingredients like aloe vera. If you're prone to prickly heat, look for a gel formulation. You can also buy aftersuns with built-in self-tanning ingredients and/or tan accelerators – a must if you're someone who adores a tan.

You can follow with a spritz of scent before you go out for the evening, but be aware that perfumes can be sensitising when they interact with sun, so shower it off before you put on your SPF in the morning. I like to spray fragrance just under my hair at the back, where it wafts when I turn my head, and also spray my beach sarongs and even my bag, to get the pleasure of the fragrance without risking a rash.

Alison's Tip

Did you know that UV light can penetrate through windows? If you're in a car, bus or lorry (particularly at the side window), a conservatory or you spend a lot of time near a window in the office, make sure you are wearing SPF, as if you were outdoors.

The ultimate fake tan

Fake tans now offer can't-tell-them-from-real results, when used in the right way. So here's my guide to your best faux glow...

Fake tans offer no protection against UV

You'll need to use your regular SPF products to protect your skin when out and about. (You can get SPF formulations with a little self-tan in now – be careful when applying these to avoid patchy application and stained palms.)

There's a self-tanner for everyone

For so many years, self-tanning products were heavy and gave orangey results, but new formulations offer can't-tell-it-from-real results.

Self-tanners are now available as sprays, mists, gels, drops and waters, so there's plenty of choice for application and texture.

Both regular self-tanners and gradual self-tanners (body lotions with a touch of self-tan, for buildable colour) are now also available in tinted versions, which are ideal if you find you miss areas because you can't see where you've applied product.

Dark skin tones can benefit from the extra glow of a self-tanner. They can be brilliant for countering ashiness or sallowness.

Self-tanners work on all skins to eliminate pallor if you've been ill or stressed, or are just fatigued.

Don't use a new self-tanner before an important event

Night before a wedding, a big date, a job interview? Have a little practice with a new self-tanner, perhaps on a casual weekend. Do be aware that there's no set standard for self-tanner; what's 'Light' in one range might be 'Medium' in another. If you were to end up darker than you'd planned, or (heaven forbid) patchy, it can just add to your stress-load. If you're using a new product for the first time, do a small section (out of sight) before you use the product all over.

Accidents shouldn't happen with today's formulas – but better safe than sorry.

Exfoliate before using self-tanner

Exfoliated skin – like a wall, sanded before painting – is the best canvas. Fake tan ingredients cling to dry, dead skin cells on thicker areas of skin, such as elbows, backs of hands, knees, ankles and wrists, so prep by removing dead skin with a suitable body/face exfoliator the night before you self-tan. (See also my tip on p.297 about 'skimming' self-tan over areas that are prone to dryness.)

If you're a tanning 'beginner', choose a tinted formula

These allow you to see where you've applied the product, for even coverage. My best tip is to check out your reflection as you apply in a full-length mirror to make sure you're applying evenly.

Don't self-tan after a bath/shower/gym session

Sweat and self-tanner don't mix, and you'll go on perspiring for some time after a bath/shower/gym session, which will make your tan patchy. If you've recently washed your hair, wrap it in a towel to stop it dripping and causing the tan to streak.

Skin must be well-moisturised so that fake tan 'takes'

Smooth lotion or butter (but not oil) into areas of dryness, especially hands, knees, elbows, wrists and feet. Allow a few minutes to sink in before applying the self-tanner itself.

I like to use disposable gloves for application

If you apply with bare hands and you're not quick at doing so, the colour can take to calluses and dry areas, so always use gloves. I find disposable gloves work better than sponge mitts. At a pinch, I'll wrap clingfilm round my hand and use that surface for application. (If you don't want to use gloves, mitts or film, you must wash your hands thoroughly with soap, immediately afterwards.)

Get naked

It's honestly the best way for even application and to avoid getting the formula on your underwear. However, if you're using a spray product, wear flip-flops because otherwise your soles will pick up self-tanner where it's misted on the floor.

Having said that... The best way to make a fake tan look truly real is to apply so it creates fake flip-flop marks on your feet, and even fake underwear marks. Don't wear your best underwear while you're doing it; keep an old set just for this – nobody will believe it's not a real tan.

Apply first to thighs, upper arms

Squirt or dollop self-tanner onto large areas of skin and massage outwards using circular strokes. When it comes to the areas tan can cling to (backs of hands, wrists, knees, ankles and heels), just drag a tiny bit of self-tan from the thighs or arms over the 'clingy' areas, for the lightest coverage. Don't hop from body part to body part; you want to be methodical: all of one leg, all the other. All of one arm, all the other.

Alison's Tip ───────────────────────

If you want to drink while you're self-tanning your face, use a straw to avoid any clown-like pale patches at the sides of your mouth.

Progressive/gradual tans can be less 'risky'

These deliver subtle, gentle colour and are a brilliant place to start if you've never self-tanned before. Some are like a body lotion with a small amount of tanning ingredient that you can build, day by day, till you achieve the desired level of bronzeness. Others come in the form of tanning drops; you use a pipette to add a couple of drops to your regular facial moisturiser or body moisturiser and smooth in as usual. There are also lightweight sprays that you can spritz on under your regular moisturiser. By next morning, you'll have a very subtle glow, which you can gradually increase until you've reached your perfect sun-kissed shade, then use every few nights (or mornings), for maintenance.

WHEN YOU'VE OVER-GLOWED

If you've stained your hands, soak them in warm water with a cup of bran and some lemon juice, then scrub with a nail brush after soaking. Body scrubs (or hand scrubs) will also help to remove excess tan, as will using a glycolic peel product. If the colour's uneven on your body, though, sometimes the best thing is to 'blur' by adding another coat of self-tan, diluted half-and-half with body lotion. You can also use body make-up or a tinted gel on areas you've missed, to disguise them.

There are no 'rules' with how much tanning ingredient is in self-tanning products and I find even the gradual tanners nowadays can contain quite high levels. I'd always do a small trial patch first to check the tanning level, before using all over.

Don't get dressed immediately

Formulations are so much better than they used to be – once upon a time it took hours of hopping around, before you could get dressed – but it's still better to stay in loose clothing after self-tanning. If you do need to get into tighter clothes, leave at least half an hour before dressing. Be aware: bedclothes and towels can take on a fake tan, so avoid sitting on your best furniture while you're waiting for your tan to dry!

Facial tanning serums are not like normal facial serums

Read the instructions! Many of them should be added in very small doses to your regular skincare, rather than smoothed all over the face – or you may go so bronzed you'll want to hide indoors for a week (it happened to a friend). Remember to blend down the neck (into your body tan) and to wash hands afterwards.

If you're self-tanning your face, apply a balm to protect your brows (and beard, for men)

You can use Vaseline, a multi-purpose balm or facial oil, stroked onto the hairs, otherwise these can pick up the self-tanner and go an unwanted shade. Take fake tanner right up to the brow-line. After you've tanned, run a slightly damp cloth over your brows and the hairline. For men with stubble, a mist tan is probably best for you. Wipe over any facial hair with a dry flannel to remove the risk of hairs turning orange.

Ask Alison: suncare Q&A

I've heard every question about tanning and self-tanning under the sun. Here are answer to some of the most frequently asked questions...

Q: I'm prone to prickly heat – what can I do?

A lot of people can't cope with the sun and heat and erupt in heinously itchy raised lumps and bumps. A tan accelerator may be a game-changer for you, because it can help prepare skin for the sun; do try it on your next holiday, or better still, from the spring onwards.

If you still find that you break out in prickly heat, do what you can to take the agony out of the situation. If you're at a bar, run ice cubes over your wrists to cool yourself down. Soak flannels and towels in cold water back in your room, and lay onto skin for relief. Be sure to take in plenty of fluids, too. And of course, you also have the option of antihistamines – speak to a pharmacist about this.

If you're someone who regularly suffers badly with prickly heat, you may want to do some homework before you book your next holiday. Ideally you want somewhere you can retreat to with air conditioning for relief, so backpacking, camping or staying in hot, humid accommodation may not be for you.

Q: How can I tan evenly? I go patchy...

Use a tan accelerator before your next holiday and you may find that changes; sometimes it means you can successfully tan your shins or tummy or other bits that stay stubbornly pale, for the first time. But your best friend may just be a self-tanner to even up the appearance of your tan – even if you're just faking it.

Q: How do I make my tan last longer?

Take your exfoliator on holiday. It will help you achieve a more even result, used regularly – and that's the key. People sometimes think that a post-holiday exfoliation will remove their tan, but that only happens if they aren't already exfoliating regularly; provided you've been scrubbing up, it will help maintain a glowing and even tan.

Keep the moisture topped up, because it's dry and flaky skin that looks dusty, giving the impression your tan is fading. Do also use a tan accelerator and choose aftersuns or post-holiday products that promise to prolong your tan with accelerators in the formula.

Q: I think I'm allergic to chemical sunscreens. What can I do?

Do some investigation into the sunscreen ingredients in your current brand, and switch to something that features different chemicals. Be sure to do a patch test, ideally on a sunny day, because you may be fine with a chemical sunscreen indoors, but find that it interacts and irritates when you expose your skin to UV light. If you're buying it for a winter sun holiday, that 'sun test' might be tricky, still patch test it on your skin beforehand, ideally on a sunny day.

Be aware, though, that it may not be the sunscreen you're sensitive to, but something else in the formula. Often, people who react to chemical sunscreens will do better with physical sunblocks, i.e. titanium dioxide and zinc oxide, which sit on the skin's surface and work by bouncing the UV light off the skin, so try switching to one of these. If you dismissed those in the past because they made you look chalky or ghostly, give them another go: many options are completely invisible as formulations have improved hugely. Natural food stores often have a wide selection of formulas which might be less reactive for you, and you'll also find them online.

Q: How do I apply make-up when I'm wearing SPF?

If you want to wear make-up in the sun, you must use a once-a-day SPF, because if you use a repeat application product, you'll mess up your make-up next time you have to reapply sunscreen. But my best advice is to switch to a self-tanner instead of make-up, to even up your skin tone just as a tinted moisturiser would. For the beach, get brows and lashes tinted before you go and you can save hassle. Or just wear a pretty sheer lipstick or tinted SPF balm, add a sweep of mascara, a touch of eyeliner pencil and do a little brow work. Add sunglasses – the best accessory ever. Save full make-up for the evening, if you really want to go to town.

Q: I get a good tan but I still tend to burn. What's going on?

Dehydrated skin will burn more readily, so if you're in a windy place, that will really affect skin's moisture level and speed up burning. (Think about what happens when you leave washing on a line on a windy day.) Start the day with a once-a-day sunscreen as protection, but if you're going on a boat, skiing, or you're on a breezy beach, top it up with a repeat-application product, which will deliver a good moisture surge that counteracts the drying effect of the wind. This is also essential if you already have dry or dehydrated skin.

Q: How do I treat peeling skin?

If you've sunburned, skin can peel off, revealing very vulnerable pink patches underneath. Whatever you do, don't tug the edges of the peeling skin to remove them. Very gentle exfoliation can be useful to remove these dead cells: first, buffer skin with a body oil, massaged all over. If you're using a salt scrub to exfoliate, dilute it half-and-half to make it gentler. Exfoliate every other day, then generously apply body cream or butter afterwards. Softly, softly, is the rule here.

Switch to a self-tanner instead of make-up for the beach, to even up your skin tone just as a tinted moisturiser would.

Beauty and beyond

"

Beauty is about the inside-out

Beauty is about the inside-out as well as the outside-in. Which means you can apply the most expensive products in the world, invest time and money in treatments, but unless you're getting enough sleep, eating well and paying attention to your overall wellbeing, you won't see all the benefits. (In fact, you might be wasting both your time and your money.) So: here are the positive steps that will ensure you not only look good, but feel great, too...

The skin is a barometer of everything else that's going on in your body. So everything you do for your body and mind – good and bad – shows up there, too. Exercise, diet, food, sleep and lifestyle all have an impact on skin, just as they do on everything you can't see.

What that also means is that something as superficial as a rash can be an indicator that something's not quite right with your overall health. I long ago realised the link between what I eat and my skin. When I was a teenager and in my early twenties, suffering from endless breakouts, I clocked that my breakouts were worse if I ate acid fruits. It wasn't the typical 'chocolate-gives-you-spots' thing; this was something that we consider very healthy which was causing the problem. Since then, I've often observed that people who go on dramatic juice fasts often tend to break out quite badly – and I don't believe you need to go to that extreme to lose weight or improve skin. My approach is essentially 'all things in moderation.'

Quite often, something like a great night's sleep or a stiff walk will leave you looking fresher than the best 'glow drops' on the market, by bringing oxygen and nutrients to the skin's surface (they will also make you feel fantastic, of course).

Eating well, in particular, making sure we get enough vitamins, essential fatty acids and our five-a-day 'rainbow' of colourful fruit and veg, shows not only in our silhouette, but also on our faces. By contrast low-fat diets can leave the skin dry, thirsty and under-nourished. As the largest organ in your body, your skin is going to show up the positive and negative aspects of your overall health. So will hair, nails and eyes (which will sparkle – or not).

So, over the next few pages, I'm going to share what I've learned about beauty from the inside out. I'm not about to recommend a diet that will help you lose weight – or put weight on; if that's an issue for you, your doctor is the best person to discuss this with. However, I can share with you what I've learned about weight management, eating healthily and exercising through my training and over my adult lifetime, and what I've shared with clients throughout my professional life.

Banish the 'd' word

When I look at someone, their weight isn't something that registers. I'd never tell someone they need to lose a few pounds, or perhaps put a few on. As far as I'm concerned, it's time to get away from the tyranny of the 'diet book', and instead, eat for health, as a priority.

If you have a friend who is always on at you about your weight, let me start by saying, to me, that isn't friendship. I don't even like it when people comment to a friend (or to me!): 'Gosh, have you lost weight?' Because implicit in that is the criticism that the person didn't look so good before. Instead, I'll compliment someone about their lipstick or their great-looking skin, or a nice haircut. I'm a great believer in 'do as you would be done by'. So, always be kind and encouraging to friends: we are more than a dress size or a suit size.

The bottom line is that we all come in different shapes and sizes, and that shape and size can change with our life stages and the natural ageing process. Media pressure, however, tells us we're meant to have the body of a 19-year-old at 55 – but please don't beat yourself up about the fact that you're not the same size as you were in your 20s and

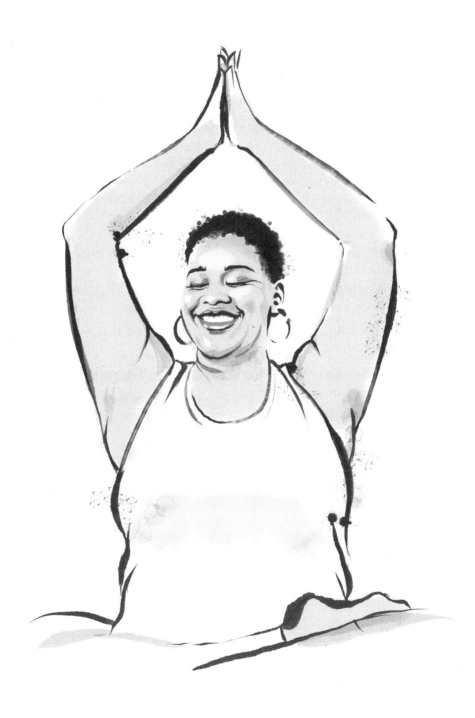

30s. Today, even men and women in their 20s and 30s already feel the pressure to have a perfect body. My very best advice to everyone is to stop comparing yourself to anyone.

That so-called 'perfection' that inspires so much envy is only possible with the right genes and a huge investment both in terms of time and money. Instead, embrace who you are and focus on doing things that make you feel good about yourself: exercising to feel healthy, taking care of your skin from top to toe so that it's smooth, silky and lovely to touch.

I'm not going to give you a blueprint for how to lose or put on weight; we're all individual, which means that a different approach works for every single one of us. But I will say: be kind to yourself, at all times. Because at the end of the day, there's just one important question: are you fit enough to enjoy the life you want to live? That's what really matters.

We are more than a dissize.

When it comes to weight, it's not helpful to set big goals

It can be a real pressure to set a specific 'goal' for a specific timeframe. Instead, start putting positive behaviours in place, and take a gradual, less stressful approach. It can help stop you falling off the wagon (and into a biscuit tin).

Ideally, don't even stand on the scales

Far preferable to me is to go by how well you feel generally, and how well your clothes are fitting. A slightly looser waistband and perhaps a face that looks a little more sculpted are more relevant than what your scales are telling you. Human beings existed without scales for millions of years! Fluid retention and the hormonal rollercoaster means that women's weight can fluctuate by a kilo or two, irrespective of what we've put in our mouths, so scales can be very depressing.

What's more, muscle weighs more than fat so if you're embarking on a health-giving fitness programme, the needle on the scale may not budge because you're simply trading muscle for fat. If you do want to weigh yourself, do so at a set time each week, at a set time of day (we're lighter in the mornings than evenings), and don't give yourself a deadline for losing (or gaining) weight.

Think in terms of nutrition, not calories

Successive generations were raised on the idea of 'calorie-counting', which means you end up feeling guilty about almost everything that you put in your mouth. Instead, learn to eat foods that are both filling and healthy: salads and vegetables, whole grains, pulses, tofu, chicken and fish.

Get in the habit of eating something healthy — a bowl of salad, a banana, a small handful of nuts — as soon as you're hungry. That's often enough to satisfy and stop you thinking about that brownie.

Keep a health journal

We often go through life on autopilot, never quite figuring out what's helping and what's not. You can use any notebook or buy one of the purpose-designed books. There are now fitness/habit tracker apps that you can use to do the same. Write in what you drink, how many glasses of water, what you eat, the exercise you do, me-time, how your mood was (good or bad), so that you can praise yourself each day, build on it for tomorrow and make those all-important connections.

A health journal is brilliant for joining up the dots between what you've been doing, lifestyle-wise, and how well you're feeling or looking. If you have a second piece of cake and feel sluggish, that's your body telling you something. If you manage to get at least five fruit and veg into your day and you realise that's given you an extra spring in your step next morning, that's great positive reinforcement. Ask yourself: what have I been doing differently that's working? and do more of it. (Or the opposite.) If 'bad' habits are impacting on how well you feel and look, take steps to change them.

We spend our lives looking after other people, but this allows you to care for yourself. Think about it: you're checking everyone around you is eating properly, making sure they sleep well, but who's doing it for you? This puts YOU firmly on the radar.

Don't eat because you're tired

Instead, have a nap or a rest. Personally, when I do consultations with clients, they do one of two things when they're exhausted from running around: put weight on, because they're reaching for the wrong foods, or lose weight because they're burning energy. Mostly, it's the former. Very often, when we're exhausted, it's sugar that we reach for, so make sure you have healthy alternatives to hand, always: fruit, grains, nuts and seeds. And make sure you've eaten a good breakfast in the morning – porridge is fab because it releases energy slowly.

Eat the rainbow

Try to get as many colours of fruit and vegetables in the space of a day as you can. It's the simplest way to make sure you get the full spectrum of vitamins and nutrients: green, orange, red and purple.

Don't go 'low-fat'

Or not unless you're doing it under medical supervision, for health reasons. Our skins (our whole bodies, in fact) need healthy fats and oils to stay plump and lubricated. When you don't get enough good fats in your diet (from foods like avocados, oily fish, nuts and seeds), skin can literally become papery, dry and appear prematurely wrinkled. Good fats are most

I'm very often tired from working night shifts on TV, so I often skip that first meal of the day because I find it hard to tell my body clock that it's breakfast-time. But if I want to drop a few pounds, the most important thing is to make myself eat porridge for breakfast. When I do eat that porridge, I'm filled up for hours and have no interest in reaching for the sugar quick-fix of a mid-morning biscuit, to keep going.

definitely *not* the body's enemy. When you buy 'low-fat' foods, they are very often loaded with sugar, instead. The 'good' oils include olive oil, avocado oil, coconut oil and sesame oil, so use these in your dressings and cooking.

Eat mindfully

We hear a lot in the media about this – because it really makes a difference! So, what is it? If you're grabbing a piece of toast as you scoot the kids into the car in the morning, or pick at snacks while watching TV, or eat while you're staring at your computer, the appetite centre in the brain simply does not register that you're eating, and therefore doesn't give the signals that you're full.

Whatever you're eating, whatever time of day or evening, set a place at table. Use a plate, knife and fork/chopsticks, whatever. Don't have the telly on in the corner, and not even the radio or music (although conversation is fine). When we focus fully on what we're putting in our mouth, we're satisfied sooner. And when we pay attention to the flavour, texture and smell of our food, that hugely boosts the pleasure factor of eating it, too.

Don't buy clothes promising yourself you're going to fit them later

In the past, I've had too-tight jeans hanging in my wardrobe, believing that would incentivise me to lose a few pounds to fit into them. Ironically, the only time I did fit into them was after I'd lost weight through illness, so that wasn't quite the positive result I was after. But in general, it's a bad idea. It's much more important to focus on positives like how well you feel, rather than squeezing into clothes that are a size too small.

Pack your own food, for out and about

Oh, the number of times I've been on the road and had to rely on what I could find in a petrol station… Happily, packed lunches are now so fashionable that there are lots of great containers out there, perfect for taking food with you on the go. If you pack your own healthy food and snacks to take to the office, on an outing or a journey, it will: a) save you money, and b) save you being tempted by unhealthy choices. Ideally, pack it the night before so it's easy to grab and you're not too rushed in the morning.

Organise yourself a 'healthy' cupboard

In a perfect world, you wouldn't let 'junk' food in the house. The easiest way to avoid over-eating unhealthy foods is not to buy them in the first place. I know perfectly well that if I have a pack of gluten-free chocolate biscuits in the cupboard, I'm not going to be able to portion them out and have one now and then; there's going to come a moment when I'm stressed and I'll eat half the packet. Best not to give them house-room in the first place, then.

This is harder when you live with other people, particularly younger people. It's particularly hard if you're sharing kitchen cupboards with the rest of the family or flatmates, with the result that you're confronted by snacks every time you open that cupboard door. Instead, can you find a cupboard in which to keep healthier, less sugary foods and snacks for yourself, so that when you open that door you're allowed to eat anything in it? And can you fill a bowl with crunchy apples and keep it on the kitchen table or next to your work station, so that you're distracted with something healthy and just a little bit sweet, before you open the cupboard?

Consider one of the healthy 'convenience food' deliveries

There's no question that home-cooked food is, in most cases, healthier than most supermarket ready meals, which are laden with hidden sugar, salt and fat. When you cook for yourself, you know exactly what you're putting in your mouth. Back in the day I did 'A' Level Domestic Science (cookery) but not everyone does a lot of cooking at school. If you missed out on that, or didn't learn at a parent's elbow, there are some great box schemes that deliver to your door all the elements of a healthy meal to make yourself – including many veggie options – with recipes and instructions. Even though they can work out slightly expensive, there's no food wastage and they can teach you cooking skills and boost your cookery confidence; you can keep the recipe cards for future use and buy the ingredients again. They're another way to ensure that you have healthy options at your fingertips, and their sheer popularity proves that this idea's working for many people. There are also many very entertaining cook-along tutorials on social media and YouTube which are free, too!

Consider a basic multivitamin/mineral supplement

A multivitamin/mineral supplement can be a sort of 'insurance policy', to make sure you have all the basics covered. Ideally, always look for food-source/natural source supplements (natural food stores are the best places to shop for these, I find, where the staff are often very knowledgeable about the products on the shelves). Failing that, look at online reviews from people who've been taking those supplements for a while. Look for high numbers of five-star reviews.

If you really feel you're deficient, your GP is your first port of call; he or she may offer a blood test to establish nutrient levels. Or you could look for a private nutritionist; shop around, and try to get recommendations from friends, because you'll have to pay for a consultation.

It may be wise for everyone to take a vitamin D supplement (available very inexpensively), as well as some kind of Essential Fatty Acid supplement, which can help with skin suppleness. If you do have weak nails or you feel like your hair's thinning, check out a specifically formulated 'skin, hair and nails' supplement. Ideally, buy from reputable companies that have been around for years and do research themselves – if you dig around on their websites, all the info is there. But be aware: vitamins aren't like scrubs or face masks that deliver instant results; it can take up to three months to start to see a difference in how skin is renewing, or nails are strengthening.

Fill yourself with vegetables first

Start a meal with a salad or soup. Load the front end of your meal with lots of healthy veg, and you'll be fuller, faster, and won't feel so like indulging in a sugar-powered dessert at the end of the meal. What you really want to avoid is getting to the table so famished that you hit the bread basket and the butter dish, and all good intentions fly out of the restaurant or kitchen window.

Sip your way to two litres a day

Drinking plenty of water is one of those positive health habits it's really worth working on: water is fantastic for hydrating skin from within, and also for keeping the digestion moving, which again shows up on the outside. Drinking more water is one free thing you can do which will make a difference that you and everyone else can see, in terms of overall bloom.

Two litres equals about eight glasses of water a day; herbal teas count towards the total, too. A lot of people struggle with that goal, so I think it's helpful to measure out your 'quota' of water at the start of the day, and either pour it into drinking bottles or into jugs in the fridge, if you're going to be at home. That takes away the guesswork.

If you've got a water bottle wherever you go – the school run, gym, the commute to work – you'll reach that target easily. Ideally, buy water bottles that are small enough to fit in your bag – if they're too heavy, you'll find any excuse not to carry them with you (especially if you haven't been a regular water drinker). I also keep a glass of water at the computer, and on my bedside.

My tip is whenever I have a tea or a coffee, I have a small glass of water as a 'chaser' (just like they do in Italy!). If I drink wine, I also always have plenty of water, too.

SMALLER PLATE, SMALLER APPETITE

When it comes to cutting down on the amount you eat, the simplest trick of all is to switch to a smaller plate. It sounds so ridiculously simple, but researchers at Cornell University and the Georgia Institute of Technology discovered that shifting from 12-in to 10-in (30cm to 25cm) plates resulted in a 22 per cent decrease in calories. If the average dinner is 800 calories, that adds up to a loss of over four kilos over a year. If you put a small piece of food on a large plate, your mind says you're eating a smaller portion, and you'll load your plate with more. If you put that same piece of food on a small plate, the brain thinks you're eating a big portion. It's extraordinary, but it works.

Alison Tip

If you want to flavour water, keep a jug in the fridge with slices of cooling cucumber or refreshing lemon. SodaStreams have massively come back into fashion, and are more environmentally friendly than shipping glass or plastic bottles of fizzy water from halfway around the world. Try diluting fruit juices with water (sparkling or still) for a refreshing juice, with half the sugar and less acid. Drinking it from a wine glass makes it feel more special too!

Think before you drink

Alcohol is fun, and relaxing – which of us hasn't felt we needed to unwind with a glass of wine after a stressful day? But for me, the key is responsible drinking. If you drink every night, you're loading up with dead calories, and this has an impact on skin (which becomes dehydrated, pale) and hair (lacklustre, dry). That's a beacon of what's happening to your whole body, as the liver tries to process the alcohol. Alcohol also affects sleep patterns; many people find that they fall asleep easily after a few drinks, but wake up in the small hours and can't get back to sleep, because the alcohol's being processed.

The way the body works is the more we have of something, the more we want it, and so drinking too much is a habit you want to nip in the bud, before it becomes a problem. Nowadays you don't need to feel deprived or left out by not drinking. There are so many delicious alternatives to alcohol (and most are far less expensive), so that you needn't ever feel you're missing out. You can get good zero-alcohol versions of many beers and wines now. Try some of the 'gin alternatives' which are appearing on the shelves. These aren't inexpensive, but often you can barely tell the difference from the real thing, with soda or tonic and a twist of lime. And my best tip here is always to drink your non-alcoholic alternatives in a great glass (a proper wine, beer or cocktail glass), so that it feels like you're enjoying something special, rather than 'depriving' yourself. Save the alcohol for special treats or nights out.

The bottom line is: all things in moderation

If someone tells you not to eat cake, I can guarantee all you'll think about is cake. Don't be a party pooper at celebrations and family events; join in the fun and get back on track with healthier eating the next day. Life's much too short not to indulge ourselves occasionally, and when we do it now and then, we appreciate it all the more. I always say: is the cake/treat worth breaking the rule for? Is it a truly fantastic piece of patisserie or a cake baked with love? In which case, have a slice and enjoy it.

Get your beauty sleep

Do you spring out of bed with a bounce in your step, or hit the snooze button and roll over? Here are the secrets of better rest – because it's not called 'beauty sleep' for nothing...

Sleep should be your No.1 beauty priority. It's free and it's absolutely central to health and wellbeing, physically and mentally – which is also why it causes so much distress when our sleeping patterns go awry. Lack of sleep does, very quickly and very visibly, show up on the outside. Dark circles. Ashiness. Wrinkles actually appear worse when we're tired. Slackness is affected by lack of sleep. Spots can worsen, too – basically, whatever your weakness is, lack of sleep will show it up and make it worse. And that's before we get to the mental health impact of sleep deprivation.

I am basically a shift worker – maybe not everyone's idea of what a shift worker is, but I quite often have to work all night and weekends presenting live TV shows, and there's no pattern to it. To be honest, in the beauty world, that's something I got used to early on: working in spas, we'd often finish at 10pm at night. There has never been a week in my life when I've gone to bed every night at bedtime and woken up at breakfast time, so I've picked up plenty of tips for kidding my body (and my brain) into getting to sleep – and staying asleep. So I completely empathise with key workers, people on farms looking after animals (who don't respect bedtimes!), or parents of children who wake up in the night (or won't get to sleep in the first place).

Draw a line under your day

It's incredibly tempting to go back to the computer and finish a project or an email when you've fed the family and got them settled, or simply fed yourself – but that's absolutely the worst thing you can do. More and more is understood about the sleep-disturbing impact of 'blue light', which is emitted by our phones, tablets, laptops and desktop computers. If you're heading back to a screen after dinner, it can be like having a jolt of caffeine, in terms of keeping yourself awake. (If it's a family Zoom call with friends and relatives, that's another thing – it's a pleasure and nobody should miss out on that, from time to time.)

After you've 'finished' your day, do something positive for yourself; listen to music, garden (when the evenings are long), water your plants, go for a walk, meet a friend. Equally, 'doing something for you' might also be taking your make-up off early, changing into comfier clothes. If you're working from home, it's especially important to make the distinction between the working day and relaxation – it'll help your brain shift down a gear. The need to be 'always on' in our society is hugely impacting sleep quality for millions of us, but the solution does require making an active effort to switch off.

Set a cut-off time for your devices

Social media algorithms are very clever things, determined to keep us scrolling and scrolling for hours at a time. Start with a ban on all devices at mealtimes; aim for eye contact and conversation rather than everyone looking at their TikTok or Instagram. And then have a 'bedtime' for all devices. If you have to put your phone in a box or somewhere else in the home to escape its magnetic power at night – well, you know what you've got to do. At the very least, turn off any notifications whose 'ping' might interrupt your sleep or winding-down time. Put your phone on 'airplane' mode; most phones allow you to programme certain numbers so that if it's a family emergency, they can still get through.

Set a cut-off point for caffeine

If you have trouble falling asleep, caffeine can be a big a factor. It's not just coffee and tea; cola drinks are made with caffeine that is a by-product of the coffee industry, and is incredibly powerful. Move the time you usually have your last cup of caffeinated drink back to early afternoon. Give it a week and see how your sleep is affected. If you're still having problems nodding off, move it earlier another hour, and so on. Basically join up the dots, till you figure out what your personal cut-off point is – and stick to it. And be aware that alcohol impacts sleep, too: it might be relaxing while we're drinking, but it can wake us up in the middle of the night as the body works to metabolise it and remove it from the body.

Eating earlier can be really helpful

You want to give your digestion as much time to settle down before you try to get to sleep. Your dinner time depends on so many factors, including a commute/how close you live to the office/whether you're trying to get kids to bed, this can be a problem. Some nights are going to be tough, but eat as early as you personally can, based on your lifestyle. If you do want to eat earlier, consider a slow cooker that basically cooks dinner while you're out – or prep food for the week on a Sunday, making dishes that can be on the table in 20 minutes.

Don't watch TV mindlessly

Don't just flop down and reach for the TV controller, at the end of the day. It's all too easy to get into the habit of passively watching that very

MAKE TIME FOR YOU

If you find you put yourself at the bottom of the list, put an entry in your diary that says, 'Me-Time'. I'm not going to prescribe what you do with that time, because it's different for all of us. In my case, it means having a shower or a bath until I've pretty much used up every drop of hot water in the tank, or looking after the animals on my farm, focusing on them, which at the same time completely switches off my brain. For you, it might be knitting. Painting. Yoga. Running. Carpentry. DIY. Jigsaws. Sudoku. Reading. Walking. Meeting a friend. You get the drill. But to quote NIKE (even though they're more about running than knitting or DIY)... Just. Do. It.

seductive screen. Add up how many hours you watched in the last week – you may be surprised. And if you do watch a lot of TV, I think you'll also be pleasantly surprised at how much time it creates in your life, when you cut down or cut it out altogether. It gives you space for some me-time.

If you don't want to give up TV, my advice is to avoid watching the news in the evening; the images and the fear-inducing stories absolutely affect sleep and dreams. Is watching a news story about a disaster or a global crisis going to enable you to DO anything about it? No. (Keep up with news stories in the morning or at lunchtime.) For the same reason, avoid watching anything scary or unpleasant, which can literally invade your sleep. It's also important to move the TV out of the bedroom, where it's just too easy to channel-surf or keep yourself awake, mindlessly viewing. With catch-up TV, there's almost nothing that you can't watch again at a future time – but if you miss those hours of sleep, you've missed them forever.

Reading paper books is good, by contrast (rather than on a screen), because it slows the brain down – but try to avoid gripping thrillers or violence, or anything that will make your adrenaline surge.

Your bedroom should be a sanctuary

Make it as restful and comfortable as budget allows. Have your lights on dimmers, and have bedside lamps, so that you can gradually reduce the light levels towards sleep-time. Buy the nicest sheets you can afford, and if your pillows are past their best, buy new ones. The test is to place a pillow over your stretched-out arm; it should stay firm and straight; if it droops, it's time to replace it. Let me tell you, by the time pillows start to flop, they're full of dust mites (which are also linked with allergies).

Have comfy throws and different textures; make your bed look beautifully inviting and you'll want to spend more time in it. (None of this need cost a fortune; supermarkets sell fantastic, high-quality bedding at very low prices now, or ask for bedlinen for your next birthday.) Keep the bedroom as tidy as you can, which cuts down on mental clutter. Make your bed in the morning – you deserve to return to a sanctuary not a mess.

Try to establish a wind-down routine

That might be going to bed at 9pm, or 10pm – whatever works for you. But try to stick with it as religiously as you can. Take a shower, or a bath; the cooling of the brain after it's been heated in a bath or shower actually helps us get to sleep. Spray your pillow and your nightclothes with a pillow mist featuring sleep-beckoning oils like lavender, vetiver, frankincense or chamomile. When you make a habit of it, those oils will actually start to trigger feelings of sleepiness, just like the smell of baking bread makes you feel hungry.

If you can't sleep, don't lie there tossing and turning

Fretting that you're not sleeping, staring at a clock that's getting later and later, can make it harder to get back to sleep. Break the cycle. And whatever you do, DON'T START LOOKING AT YOUR PHONE. (Yes, those are 'bossy' capitals.) Try these instead:

- Get up and make yourself a herbal tea or a milky drink (no caffeine).

- Mist a hankie or tissue with pillow spray and sniff it, or put some soothing essential oils in a diffuser (lavender, vetiver, chamomile, frankincense, as before – or whatever blend works for you; there are many, many sleep-beckoning essential oil blends out there now).

- Read a relaxing book.

- Listen to a mindfulness/sleep podcast.

- Listen to 'white noise' (you can find apps for this), such as breaking waves on a shore, thunderstorms, leaves rustling in trees... Identify what works for you and play it when you're having trouble sleeping. (And if you share a bed with someone, get some headphones.)

HOW TO SLEEP THROUGH THE MENOPAUSE

If you have sailed through the menopause with undisturbed sleep, congratulations. More than that, I'm quite envious; I went through an absolutely terrible menopause myself, during which I didn't sleep for more than 40 consecutive minutes, for over five years (not to mention the hot flushes every few minutes, which I had to deal with on live television); I wasn't allowed medication, because of conflicts with other prescriptions – so I've been there, done that and wrung out the nightie. You might be luckier; if you're experiencing problems, you can always consult your GP.

If you overheat in bed, sleep on a towel

A big, thick fluffy towel will absorb the sweat. It needs to be a generous bath sheet; tuck it under your pillow and smooth it all the way down to where your heels rest.

Try a USB plug-in desk fan

Plug this into a USB charger on your bedside table; these are very quiet fans and the air flow can be all you need to feel cooler, even if it's only directed at your face and neck.

Change your bedlinen

Linen sheets and pillowcases are coolest. If you wake up and you're hot, flip your pillow over to the cool side.

If you're sweating a lot, drink water with electrolytes

Especially if you start to notice a lot of headaches, which is a sign of dehydration. Good natural electrolytes are (dairy) milk or coconut water, or use the soluble sachets of electrolytes you can pick up in the pharmacy.

Go and cool down

If you're really too hot, go and open the freezer door; maybe keep a flannel in there that you can use to cool yourself down. Or open the back door. Basically, if you can't cool down in bed, go somewhere else to take the temperature down – and the bed will have cooled down by the time you get back in, too, offering relief.

Keep your moisturiser by the bed

If you overheat, your face products will literally be sweated into the pillow, and a dollop of moisturiser on the face in the middle of the night can feel very soothing and cooling.

Don't panic!

Try to accept the little sleep you get and be thankful you will get to sleep again. Clock-watching and panicking only make it worse. Five or six sets of 40-minute sleeps is a lot more than one or two, because you have started worrying in the night.

THE TRICK OF
A TREAT

To motivate yourself, schedule in regular rewards. Treating yourself to a massage or a facial every couple of months, for example, can be a brilliant way to pat yourself on the back (or rather, having someone else pat you on the back – literally). It might sound like kid's stuff, but making a chart and sticking it on the fridge, then ticking off the days you work out or do your weights or flexibility training is an incredibly powerful motivation, especially if you earmark a 'reward' in advance.

Move it!

Optimum fitness doesn't mean being able to run a marathon or climb Kilimanjaro. It means being flexible enough, strong enough and with enough stamina to do everything we'd like to do, in a 'normal' life…

Fitness used to be built into daily life. Back in the day, the idea of a day out for many families was to go for a walk in the countryside or a stroll along the beach. We tended to go from A to B on foot more in daily life, walking or cycling to work locally etc. Now we have cars, plentiful public transport and Uber and life is just so darned 'convenient' that we have to make an effort to exercise, rather than weave it into our lives. So: it's time to get off that couch, if you haven't already embraced a fitter way of life. Ideally, you want to incorporate exercise in easy ways that cover these three 'pillars' of fitness:

1. RESISTANCE

This is about muscle strength. As we age, muscle strength dips dramatically – but it doesn't have to. And you don't need to sign up for a gym or make a big investment in home gym equipment (which generally tends to end up as a very expensive clothes horse, in my experience). You can use stretchy rubber bands and/or lift light weights (tins of baked beans will do, if you don't have weights to hand!), to improve muscle tone and strength.

Your own body weight offers resistance too; little things like gentle squats while you're waiting for the kettle to boil, or doing standing press-ups against a wall, are helpful. Stepping up and down on the bottom stair, while holding the banisters for stability, can mirror what you'd do in a gym class. Carrying shopping back from the shops (provided you balance your shopping bags and walk with your shoulders back) is great for strengthening upper arms.

2. FLEXIBILITY AND BALANCE

You don't need to be able to do the splits, but flexibility's so vital – for men and for women – to help avoid aches and pains and muscle injury, which can stop you doing things you enjoy. Flexible people tend to have a much better sense of balance, too, which can help you avoid falls in later life.

Pilates and yoga are very beneficial for flexibility, balance and strength. The fact that yoga and Pilates have literally millions of devotees all over the world says a lot. Again, you don't even need to leave home to do them; there are so many classes offered online, at all levels from beginner to expert. This makes it affordable, you can try out different teachers, and no-one will see if you can't touch your toes; you can find classes that start with as little as 20 minutes, which is great as you ease yourself into it. Once you've built up your confidence you can then find local classes, which is a chance to socialise as well as get fitter. You'll find that yoga, Pilates and stretching generally works wonders on posture (which is especially important if you are a desk-worker) – and improved posture can, in turn, almost magically take years off your appearance, too.

One last point on stretching: because so many of us spend hours at the computer each day, it's important to stand up and do some stretching exercises for arms, legs, necks and backs at regular points in the day, to unkink muscles. Walk around every hour or so, or set a timer to leave the desk for 5–10 minutes. Again, you can find specialist at-desk/post-desk exercises, online. It's another case of: Just. Do. Them.

3. STAMINA

The final exercise 'must' is to find an aerobic exercise that you enjoy and will do regularly – if you don't want anything more strenuous than walking, that's fine. Aerobic exercise has so many benefits: it reduces the risk of obesity, high blood pressure, heart disease, type 2 diabetes, stroke and even some kinds of cancer. More reasons to do it are that weight-bearing aerobic exercise (e.g. walking, running and skipping), help reduce your risk of osteoporosis. What's not to love about that?

The accepted recommendation for optimum health is to notch up at least 10,000 steps a day. And the chances are, info about how many steps you're already doing each day is literally at your fingertips. You don't need a FitBit to track your steps; the Health app on your phone has, perhaps even without you knowing it, been counting your steps since you got your phone. It came as a surprise to me, too, when a friend told me – but it's just the nudge that many of us need to become a bit self-competitive and try (gradually) to build in more activity to our days.

The NHS 'Couch to 5K' app has a free nine-week programme offering podcasts, coaching and progress-tracking, if you are new to aerobic exercise. It starts with a brisk five-minute walk, and then progresses by alternating walking and running, with lots of rest days in between. Many, many people have surprised themselves through using this app, and have jogged further than they thought possible. It's accompanied by a five-week Strength and Flex plan, to improve flexibility and strength, both of which will help your running or jogging.

The bonus? A nice, rosy glow to your cheeks, without a smidgen of blusher required. And a self-satisfied note in your health journal about the number of steps you've managed today.

Mindfulness and meditation

I recommend that you make mindfulness and meditation as much a part of your routine as putting on make-up or shaving.

Mindfulness isn't a new-fangled thing; it's something people have practised for millennia, but we need it more than ever, because the endless distractions in our daily lives have our thoughts dancing all over the place. We multitask, we multiscreen, so it's no wonder we feel frazzled and even burned-out, at times. The mental imbalance that our crazy lives bring about can be picked up by the body, leading to all sorts of illnesses and disorders, which is why it's so, so important to do something positive for our mental wellbeing, on a regular basis. And I can put my hand on my heart and say: when you take even just three minutes to practise mindfulness, it will give you much more than three minutes BACK in your day, in terms of how much calmer and more focused you feel.

The essence of mindfulness is about finding time in each day when you're doing something but NOT thinking about something else. When you're dropping the kids off, you focus on dropping the kids off – not the list of groceries you're about to pick up from the supermarket. When you're drinking a coffee, you're focusing on the taste, the temperature, the feel of the coffee on your tongue, not thinking about the call you've got to make in 15 minutes. You can even be mindful when washing-up!

There's a book I recommend to clients, family and friends and I'm going to recommend it to you: *Mindfulness: A Practical Guide to Finding Peace in a Frantic World*. The title just says it all, doesn't it? This book is written by Professor Mark Williams and an award-winning journalist, Dr Danny Penman, who codeveloped Cognitive Behaviour Therapy (CBT). They're the real deal. They also have an app with an eight-week mindfulness programme.

You can also learn mindfulness online, via courses, as well as face-to-face at wellbeing centres or meditation centres. Some large organisations put on courses for their workforce. But however you choose to learn mindfulness, I can't recommend too highly that you find a place for it in your day.

Alison's Tip ———————————

Try a car park meditation. When you arrive somewhere, don't rush to get out of the car and get on with your life. Take three minutes for yourself. Think mindfully about your feet, resting on the floor. Take some deep breaths. Calm your mind. Whatever you do next, you'll do it with more purpose and serenity than if you dash, dash, dash. Like all forms of meditation, it magically expands time.

Ask Alison: self-care Q&A

Q: I don't have enough time to exercise – what can I do?

Everyone thinks they don't have enough time for exercising, but it's about prioritising and rearranging life to make time. This isn't something you do 24 hours a day; I'm asking you to put aside half an hour in that 24 hours for *yourself*. The average person watches more than three hours of TV a day; watch half an hour's less telly, and get out there. But also add in bite-sized chunks of exercise, to up your activity rate. Walk to work, rather than take public transport, if you can, or at least do some of the journey on foot. Get off the bus a stop earlier. When you're waiting for the kettle to boil, do some stretching, or just lift a couple of baked bean cans, like light weights, to give your arms a workout. Do some squats, jog on the spot – this is about shifting to an active mindset. And 'audition' various kinds of exercise – walking (perhaps with a friend or a walking club), trampolining, swimming, Zumba, dance classes – to find the one you most enjoy, and which you'll look forward to. I promise you'll find the time.

Q: I think I will find meditation boring...

You don't have to spend lots of time sitting cross-legged, reciting a mantra, to meditate. You can close your eyes and do some breathing exercises when you're waiting for a train or the checkout in a supermarket. Try counting to three as you breathe in, counting to four to hold, and then five to breathe out – it works. Simply try to become mindful about what it is you're doing. If you're walking, focus on walking, rather than filling your head with To Do lists. (Try the walking meditations on calm.com, if you need guidance.) Even if you can't find time or don't want to 'formally' meditate every day, try to be 'in the moment' as much as possible, and I promise you'll clear a huge amount of head-clutter. Sometimes it's as simple as looking up from your screen and really taking in the sky, or noticing and really observing flowers or trees. Perhaps for you it's seeing the joy in child's face, or an animal's, and borrowing that smile. Notice how much calmer you feel afterwards, which will help motivate you to do it again and again.

Q: I don't have enough money to join a gym or buy exercise gear – any suggestions?

Nobody's going to charge you for walking around the block. If you don't like to walk alone (and women can sometimes feel vulnerable doing this without a dog), try to find a 'walking buddy'. I don't like walking in the countryside after dark, so you know what I do? I drive to the nearest town centre and walk around under the street lights in the heart of town, window-shopping as I go, with my dogs.

Join a rambling or walking group; these are often advertised locally. Beyond lacing up your trainers and walking, there are literally hundreds of free or inexpensive online classes that you can take, via a computer, whether it's PE with Joe Wicks or a yoga class streamed from Bali.

When it comes to exercise gear, so many places now sell incredibly affordable exercise clothing. But you may not need special kit; you may well be able to get away with the kind of loose clothing you wear for relaxing at home, as long as you're not going to trip over the hem of your trousers!

There really are no more excuses. You can sit on the couch and look at programmes about people's houses, or you can walk around your neighbourhood and look at real houses. You can watch programmes about nature and the countryside – or you can get off the sofa and get out there, to experience it for yourself. It's that simple!

Q: I need someone to help motivate me. Where should I turn?

A diet and/or an exercise buddy is great, if you're not strongly motivated on your own. Who do you know who would also like to get a bit healthier? I can absolutely promise you'll have someone in your life, probably more than one person, if you think about it. You want someone you can ring up and ask, 'Would you like to come out for a walk?' Or who you can drive somewhere with to get out in nature, with a healthy packed lunch, to turn a day out into something positive for your health. You can even take that a stage further, if you're trying to lose weight, WhatsApping pictures of your healthy meal or positively reinforcing the things each of you does to get fitter, become healthier.

Q: What can I do if bad knees are stopping me from exercising?

Almost everyone's got some form of injury or weakness. (Knees are definitely my weak point.) If you can't go running, that doesn't stop you exercising. Walk, instead! Cycling is another gentler alternative, or swimming, or Pilates, which offers exercises for strengthening the muscles either side of the knee to take the pressure off the knee joint.

Q: When it comes to eating well, I start with good intentions and then slip up. How can I change that?

'Get back on the horse,' as they say. Nobody's perfect. Tomorrow is another day, so don't use it as an excuse but don't beat yourself up about it, either. And if you really can't bear to give up certain indulgences, then consider a diet that allows you to have 'treat days', like a 5:2 or a 6:1 diet, so that you don't feel deprived and want to throw in the towel over what feels like a cake-free, Brie-free, fun-free future.

The feel-good factor

Things you can do to make yourself feel better, fast...

We all have slumps. Moments when our get-up-and-go has got-up-and-gone. Times when we need a boost. When that happens, try any or all of these 100 per cent free pick-me-ups.

The secret is to just do something different. Even just turning around your desk, sitting in a different chair in the lounge, turning the radio or TV off and listening to bird sound can change your outlook.

1. **Drink a glass of water.** Often being dehydrated can make us feel stressed, and simply rehydrating with a glass of water is an amazing quick fix.

2. **Take a catnap.** And don't feel guilty about it.

3. **Make a positive move towards a good sleep plan.** Tidy your bedroom so it's more of a sanctuary; hang up the clothes that are over the back of the chair and lay out your bedtime beauty products.

4. **Pay someone a compliment.** It feels SO good to say to someone, 'Your hair looks great' or 'I love that colour on you.' As nice as, if not better than, receiving a compliment!

5. **Put on a little make-up.** A touch of lipstick. A smidge of light-reflective concealer on dark circles. An extra coat of mascara, to show off your eyes.

6. **Have a shave or trim your facial hair.** The masculine equivalent of putting on make-up, for a quick pick-you-up to make you feel more groomed, instantly.

7. **Go for a walk.** If you just keep doing what you're doing, you'll keep feeling like you're feeling and won't get motivated.

8. **Go to your kitchen and eat something healthy/nourishing.** Do it now, before you hit the cake, biscuits and crisps because you're famished.

An apple a day, for instance, is packed with quercetin, and it's not just an Old Wives' Tale: it really does help to keep the doctor away.

9. **Meditate for five minutes.**

10. **Flip your parting over.** Hey, presto, instant new look! Or zhoosh some dry shampoo through your hair.

11. **Put on some uplifting music and dance to the next track.** Smile while you're doing it, which releases endorphins – and remember, nobody can see you!

12. **Do a bit of decluttering.** Sort out your make-up bag or your travel beauty/grooming kit. Creating order out of chaos is a real mood-booster.

13. **Change out of your 'comfy' clothes.** Yes, it's nice to change into something slouchy when we get home from work or at the end of a hard day, but when we're mooching around in sweatpants or PJs and slippers all day, the energy-boost of putting on something with a waistband and a proper shoulder and buttons can completely shake up how we feel.

14. **Brush your hair.**

15. **Burn some uplifting essential oils.** Citrus notes like lime, grapefruit and mandarin are all wonderfully sense-awakening.

16. **Paint your nails.**

17. **Go to your wardrobe and put together some new combinations.** There. Saved yourself a shopping trip.

18. **Do a yoga pose.** When you're practising yoga, there's almost always one pose that becomes a favourite. Do it now!

19. **Phone a friend.** An actual call, not a comment on Facebook or Instagram. We thrive on human connection.

20. **Spray on a favourite fragrance.** We should all have something in our fragrance wardrobe that is just energy-in-a-bottle.

A last word

My goal, with everything within the covers of this book, has been to make beauty and wellbeing accessible, positive and hugely enjoyable for you. I hope you've snuggled up on a sofa somewhere or lazed on a sun lounger to read it, carving time out for yourself – that well-deserved, much-needed TLC that is so, so important.

My whole mission in life has been to demystify grooming, beauty and wellness, signposting men and women to techniques and products that really work. I truly want you to feel good about yourself, have a beauty or grooming routine that you love, and to live as balanced and healthy life as our crazy world allows, so what you've read in this book is the insider advice that I've shared with countless beauty brands and private clients, over the years. I've tried to cover everything I've ever been asked by viewers, too, whether I happened to be coming out of a loo, waking up from an anaesthetic, or via social media.

So if I've encouraged you to take up a Zoom yoga class, shown you where to sweep your blusher so that it takes off five years or nudged you in the direction of your optimum skincare routine, that's my job done.

And now, armed with everything I've shared in this book, it's over to you...

With thanks

To my family, both human and animal, who like to stay in the background and keep me grounded – especially my brother Mark. We make a great team at home and at work.

All at alisonyoungbeauty.com and Alison Young Social, Broadcasting and Consulting HQ, who I probably drive mad at the strange and antisocial hours of the day and night when my brain goes into overdrive! Thank you for your patience, support and loyalty. Super special mention to the multitalented, loyal and long-suffering Jade (15 years and counting!) who works as hard as me and longer hours!

The glam squad – my darling Frankie, my best friend and hairdresser of 35 years. No one does blonde like you! June from Makeup–Junkies International Ltd for all my shoot hair and make-up looks, but most importantly our laughs, days off and holidays! Thanks to Lezlie and Rose (Instagram @LezlieandRose), photographers for the magical shoot for this book and so many others too. Thanks too to Jillie Murphy (JillieMurphy.com) for styling without even needing to meet (lockdown) before the shoot and getting it bang on. Also, thanks to Steve Gardner for shoot co-ordination and website design.

To PR Nancy Brady of @NBPR who finally got her way, as this book was her idea, along with the team at Vermilion. Thanks to Susanna, Emma, Leah, Nikki, Ed, Adelaide, Sarah, Caroline and all who helped make this book happen and who made this a much more pleasant process than I imagined, albeit hard work. Particular thanks to the amazing legend, the like-minded Josephine Fairley, who translated my beauty knowledge (and rants!) into decipherable English, and had the nerve to say, 'Enough, Alison, that's too much detail! That's for your next book...'

Index

Page references in *italics* indicate images.

For further information, free tutorials and live Q&As, go to Alison's website and follow her on Instagram, Twitter, Facebook and YouTube:

alisonyoungbeauty.com

 instagram.com/aliyoungbeauty   facebook.com/aliyoungbeauty

twitter.com/aliyoungbeauty   YouTube.com/aliyoungbeauty

1

Vermilion, an imprint of Ebury Publishing,
20 Vauxhall Bridge Road,
London SW1V 2SA

Vermilion is part of the Penguin Random House group of companies whose addresses can be found at global.penguinrandomhouse.com

 Penguin
Random House
UK

Text © Alison Young Limited ® 2021
Illustrations © Adelaide Leeder 2021

Alison Young has asserted her right to be identified as the author of this Work in accordance with the Copyright, Designs and Patents Act 1988

First published by Vermilion in 2021

www.penguin.co.uk

A CIP catalogue record for this book is available from the British Library

Design: Nic & Lou; Ed Pickford

ISBN 9781785043420

ALISON YOUNG and the 35 YEARS OF QUALIFIED BEAUTY EXPERIENCE ALISON YOUNG TRIED & TRUSTED logo are registered trademarks licensed to Alison Young.

PRINTED AND BOUND IN GREAT BRITAIN BY CLAYS LTD, ELCOGRAF S.P.A.

THE AUTHORISED REPRESENTATIVE IN THE EEA IS PENGUIN RANDOM HOUSE IRELAND, MORRISON CHAMBERS, 32 NASSAU STREET, DUBLIN D02 YH68.

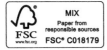

Penguin Random House is committed to a sustainable future for our business, our readers and our planet. This book is made from Forest Stewardship Council® certified paper.